your pregnancy™

ck Guide

N... ...eight Management

your
pregnancy™
Quick Guide

Nutrition and Weight Management

*What You Need to Know about
Eating Right and Staying Fit
during Your Pregnancy*

Glade B. Curtis, M.D., M.P.H., OB/GYN
Judith Schuler, M.S.

Da Capo
∞
LIFE
LONG

A Member of the Perseus Books Group

Copyright 2004 © by Glade B. Curtis and Judith Schuler

Text design by Brent Wilcox
Set in 11.5-point Minion by the Perseus Books Group

Library of Congress Cataloging-in-Publication Data

Curtis, Glade B.
    Your pregnancy quick guide to nutrition and weight management : what you need to know about eating right and staying fit during your pregnancy / Glade B. Curtis and Judith Schuler.
        p.   cm.
    Includes index.
    ISBN 0-7382-0954-6 (pbk.: alk. paper)
    1. Pregnancy—Nutritional aspects—Popular works.   2. Pregnant women—weight gain—Popular works.   3. Pregnant women—Health and hygiene—Popular works.   I. Schuler, Judith.   II. Title.
RG559.C87 2004
618.2'42—dc22

                                                                                    2004010546

First Da Capo Press printing 2004

Published by Da Capo Press
A Member of the Perseus Books Group
www.dacapopress.com

Da Capo Press books are available at special discounts for bulk purchases in the U.S. by corporations, institutions, and other organizations. For more information, please contact the Special Markets Department at the Perseus Books Group, 11 Cambridge Center, Cambridge, MA 02142, or call (800) 255-1514 or (617) 252-5298, or e-mail special.markets@perseusbooks.com.

1 2 3 4 5 6 7 8 9—08 07 06 05 04

Find It Fast!

Part I: Nutrition

Good nutrition for a mother-to-be is one of the most important keys to having a healthy baby. When you eat wisely and nutritiously, your growing baby gets the nutrients it needs to develop and to grow healthy.

Have you heard the saying, "A pregnant woman is eating for two?" It's true, you are eating for two—yourself and your baby—but you don't have to eat *twice* as much! It's more important to eat healthfully.

Some women have the misconception they can eat anything they want, and as much as they want, during pregnancy. But the truth is, if you're average weight when you begin pregnancy, you only need to eat about 300 extra calories a day for good nutrition for you *and* your baby. That's not a lot of food—you can add those extra calories by eating one 8-ounce carton of lowfat flavored yogurt and a medium apple!

The baby growing inside you has many nutritional needs—needs *you* must meet through the foods you choose. A pregnant woman who eats a healthy diet during pregnancy is much more likely to give birth to a healthy baby. Eating well reduces your risk of pregnancy complications and limits some pregnancy side effects.

Some General Guidelines

- Eating healthfully, exercising and controlling your weight during pregnancy go a long way toward giving your baby a healthy start in life.
- The foods you eat help your baby develop and grow—your baby gets the nutrients it needs from your blood.
- By eating healthfully, you provide the baby with the nutrients it needs to build its bones and organs.
- You can meet most pregnancy nutrition needs by eating a well-balanced, varied diet.
- The *quality* of your calories is important—if you eat a food in it's natural state, it's better for you than if it is processed and comes from a can or a box.
- Some women have the false idea they can eat all they want during pregnancy. Most women can't!
- Controlling your weight (not gaining too much weight but gaining enough) makes sure your developing baby gets the nutrients it needs.
- Don't gain more weight than your doctor recommends during your pregnancy—it can make you uncomfortable, and it may be harder to lose the extra pounds after baby is born.
- Gaining too much weight can cause problems during delivery because your baby may be very large.
- Eat frequent, small meals during the day to supply better nutrition to your growing baby.

- If you eat only three large meals, nutrient levels rise and fall during the day, which isn't as good for the growing baby.
- Eating small meals frequently gives you more stable nutrient levels and can also help avoid some problems, such as heartburn and indigestion.
- One study showed 95% of the women who had good-to-excellent diets during pregnancy delivered babies in good-to-excellent health.
- One of your main goals in pregnancy is to have the healthiest baby you can. Your nutrition during pregnancy has a great impact on your baby's health.
- To help you determine if you are choosing healthy foods, buy a book that lists the nutritional content of many foods. There are many available; check your bookstore.
- Reading labels on various food packages can also tell you a lot. If you haven't done this before, try it. You'll learn a great deal about the foods you eat, and it will help you eat healthfully.

Fasting—A Practice to Avoid

- Some religions have days of fasting and abstinence.
- With *fasting,* you eat very little or nothing at all during the day. With *abstinence,* you abstain from various foods, such as meat, for the entire day.

- A pregnant woman should *never* fast.
- Abstinence from meat or other specific foods is OK as long as you get the nutrients you need from other sources during the period of abstinence.

What Should I Eat?

You may be wondering what kinds of foods to eat and what to omit from your eating plan during pregnancy. The chart below offers you some general guidance. We discuss specific details later in this book.

Foods to Eat	Minimum Servings per Day
Dark green or dark yellow fruits and vegetables	1
Vitamin-C fruits and vegetables, such as tomatoes and citrus	2
Other fruits and vegetables	4
Whole-grain breads and cereals	6
Dairy products, including milk	4
Protein sources (meat, poultry, eggs, fish)	2
Dried beans and peas, seeds and nuts	2

Foods to Eat in Moderation

Caffeine	200mg
Fat	limited amounts
Sugar	limited amounts

Foods to Avoid

Anything containing alcohol
Food additives, when possible

Can I eat all I want during pregnancy?

Some women have the wrong idea about eating when they're pregnant. Unfortunately, most women *cannot* eat all they want during pregnancy—you may not be able to either. Eat wisely. Don't gain more weight than your doctor recommends, which is usually 25 to 35 pounds for the average-weight woman. Your doctor will give you a target weight gain for your entire pregnancy.

Singapore Swing

2 ounces fruit-flavored sorbet
5 ounces orange juice
dash of lime juice
Mix all ingredients in a cocktail shaker or blender. Serve in a martini glass, garnished with orange slices.

A Warning about Alcohol

We know a lot about how alcohol can affect pregnancy. Studies show a woman's use of alcohol during pregnancy may affect her child's IQ, attention span and learning ability.

- Most experts believe the safest approach to alcohol use during pregnancy is *no use at all.*

- That's the reason alcoholic beverages in the United States carry warning labels similar to those on cigarette packages.
- Alcohol crosses the placenta and directly affects your baby.
- Moderate drinking has been linked to an increased chance of miscarriage.
- Drinking a lot during pregnancy can also result in birth defects in the baby.
- Heavy drinking during pregnancy can cause fetal alcohol syndrome (FAS) or fetal alcohol exposure (FAE).
- FAS babies are usually small, before and after birth. Birth defects can appear in limbs, the heart and facial features.
- Children may have speech defects.
- Later in life, the child may have behavioral problems.
- Taking drugs with alcohol increases the chances of damage to a baby. Analgesics, antidepressants and anticonvulsants cause the most concern.
- Some researchers have even suggested heavy alcohol use by the baby's father before conception may result in problems.
- You also need to be very careful about over-the-counter cough and cold remedies you may use. Many contain alcohol—some as much as 25%!

I don't drink that much alcohol. Can't I have a glass of wine with dinner?

We advise you to avoid *all* alcohol during your pregnancy. Research has not indicated a "safe" alcohol-intake level. To protect your baby, make water, milk and juice your drinks of choice during pregnancy.

Alcohol in Cooking

Most pregnant women know they should avoid alcohol during pregnancy but what about recipes that call for alcohol? A good rule of thumb is it's probably OK to eat a food that contains alcohol if it has been baked or simmered for at least 1 hour. Cooking for that length of time evaporates most of the alcohol content.

Food-Group Recommendations

To get the nutrition you need during your pregnancy, make good food choices. Eat the recommended number of servings from each food group every day. (See the discussions that follow.)

- Eating the right foods, in the correct amounts, takes planning.

- Some foods contain more than one nutrient. For example, yogurt and cheese provide calcium and protein. One food fills two requirements!

- Choose foods high in vitamins and minerals, especially iron, calcium, magnesium, folic acid and zinc. We give you some food choices for these vitamins and minerals in later discussions.

- Taking your prenatal vitamin is important, but you also need to eat vitamin-rich foods. Don't expect your vitamin to provide all the minerals and vitamins you and your baby need—it's *not* a substitute for food.

- Always read food labels—they contain lots of different types of information.

- Labels will help you see what foods are good for you and which ones you should avoid or eat only once in awhile.

- If you have questions or concerns, discuss your nutrition plan with your doctor or a registered dietitian.

- Foods high in nutrients are good choices. Choose foods that provide a lot of nutrients but not very many calories. One example of this kind of food is fruits and vegetables—they provide a lot of vitamins and minerals but are not usually high in calories.

Nutrients You Need and Where You Can Find Them

This chart shows you where to get the various nutrients that you should be eating every day during your pregnancy. We discuss all the food groups in the sections that follow, which will help you make good food choices.

Nutrient (Daily Requirement)	Food Sources
Calcium (1200mg)	Dairy products, dark leafy vegetables, dried beans, peas, tofu, sardines, fortified whole-grain products
Folic acid (0.4mg)	Liver, dried beans and peas, eggs, broccoli, oranges, orange juice, dark leafy vegetables, legumes, nuts, fortified whole-grain products
Iron (30mg)	Fish, liver, lean red meat, poultry, egg yolks, nuts, dried beans, peas, dark leafy vegetables, dried fruit, fortified whole-grain products
Magnesium (320mg)	Dried beans, peas, cocoa, fish, fortified whole-grain products, nuts, dark leafy vegetables
Vitamin A (770mcg)	Carrots, dark leafy vegetables, sweet potatoes
Vitamin B_6 (2.2mg)	Whole-grain products, liver, meat, bananas, nuts, beans, legumes
Vitamin C (85mg)	Citrus, broccoli, tomatoes
Vitamin E (10mg)	Milk, eggs, meats, fish, cereals, leafy vegetables, vegetable oils, fortified whole-grain products, nuts, beans, legumes
Zinc (15mg)	Fish, meat, nuts, milk, dried beans, peas

Daily Recommendations

Below is a list of the various food groups, and amounts from each, that you need *every* day. We discuss these in detail following this section.

Daily Food-Group Servings

Food Group	Daily Servings
Dairy products	4
Meats and other protein sources	2 to 4
Vegetables	4
Fruits	3 to 4
Bread, cereal, pasta, rice	6 to 11
Fats, sweets and other "empty" calories	2 to 3

Understanding Serving Sizes

- After reading about your nutrition requirements, you may believe it'll be difficult to eat all the portions you need for the health of your growing baby.
- You may not understand what a "portion" or "serving" is.
- It is hard to understand how much food is enough or too much. For example, a large bagel can actually be *four* to *five* grain servings!
- If you have access to a computer, check out the USDA's website *www.cnpp.usda.gov;* it lists serving portions.

- If you can't get to a computer, ask your doctor for some nutrition handouts.

Dairy Products

You need at least 4 servings every day of various dairy products. These products contain calcium, which is important for you and your growing baby.

- Read food labels for information on the calcium content of a food.
- If you want to limit the fat content of dairy products, choose skim milk and lowfat and fatfree products. There are quite a few on the market today.
- Calcium content is not affected in lowfat or fatfree dairy products.
- Foods you might choose from this group, and their serving sizes, include:
  - ~ ¾ cup cottage cheese
  - ~ 2 ounces processed cheese (such as American cheese)
  - ~ 1 ounce hard cheese (such as Parmesan or Romano)
  - ~ 1 cup pudding or custard
  - ~ 1 8-ounce glass of milk (whole, 2%, 1%, skim)
  - ~ 1½ ounces natural cheese (such as cheddar)
  - ~ 1 cup yogurt
- Also see the discussion of calcium on page 27.

I know dairy products are a good source of calcium, but I've heard there are some milk products I should avoid. Is this true?

There are some foods made from milk that we would advise you not to eat. These include unpasteurized milk and any foods made from unpasteurized milk. Also avoid soft cheeses, such as Brie, Camembert, feta and Roquefort. These products are a common source of a form of food poisoning called *listeriosis.* We discuss listeriosis on page 56.

Protein Sources

Pregnancy increases your protein needs. Protein is very important to the healthy growth and development of your baby. Protein contains amino acids. Amino acids are critical to the growth and repair of the embryo/fetus, placenta, uterus and breasts. You need about 6 to 7 ounces of protein every day; this is about twice the amount recommended for women who are not pregnant.

- Read labels to find the protein content for various foods, and keep a running total for each day.
- Many protein sources are high in fat.
- If you need to watch your calories, choose skinless chicken and turkey, scrod, ground turkey and lowfat (1%) or skim milk.

- Eat foods that contain choline and docosahexaenoic acid (DHA).
- Choline and DHA help build baby's brain cells during fetal development and breastfeeding.
- Choline is found in milk, eggs, peanuts, whole-wheat bread and beef.
- DHA is found in fish, egg yolks, poultry, meat, canola oil, walnuts and wheat germ.
- If you eat foods that contain choline and DHA during pregnancy and while you're breastfeeding, you pass these important nutrients along to baby.
- Foods you might choose from the protein group, and their serving sizes, include:
  ~ 2 tablespoons peanut butter
  ~ ½ to 1 cup cooked dried beans (check out the type of bean you are interested in)
  ~ 2 to 4 ounces cooked meat
  ~ 1 egg
  ~ 1 ounce cheese
  ~ 1 ounce nuts
  ~ 8 ounces milk
  ~ 1 ounce tuna, packed in water (limit yourself to 6 ounces of canned tuna a week; see the discussion of fish that begins on page 20)
  ~ 8 ounces yogurt

I really love protein foods that have a lot of fat, like bacon and cheeses. What can I substitute for them?

Choose foods that are high in protein but low in fat. There are many lowfat and fatfree cheeses on the market today. You can even find bacon substitutes, which taste very good. You'll probably be surprised at the variety of lowfat or fatfree foods now available. That's why we encourage you to read food labels—you can learn a lot!

Fruits and Vegetables

Fruits and vegetables are important in your nutrition plan because they are excellent sources of vitamins, minerals and fiber. You need 4 servings of vegetables and at least 3 servings of fruit each day.

- Check a nutritional guide for information about a particular fruit or vegetable if you have questions.
- Eating a variety of fruits and vegetables supplies you with iron, folic acid, calcium, fiber and vitamin C.
- Because they change with the seasons, fruits and vegetables are a great way to add variety to your menu.
- Eat a lot of different types of vegetables—it shouldn't be hard. Green leafy veggies, such as spinach and broccoli, contain different nutrients than orange vegetables, such as yams and carrots.

- Eat at least one leafy, green or deep-yellow vegetable a day for extra iron, fiber and folic acid.
- When choosing lettuce, darker is better. Romaine and spinach have a lot of vitamin A and folic acid. Iceberg lettuce has the most fiber and is a good source of potassium. Arugula and leaf lettuce add texture and vitamins A and C.
- Include one or two servings each day of a fruit rich in vitamin C, such as grapefruit juice or orange slices.
- Have fresh fruits when possible, and drink 100% juice instead of "fruit drinks."
- Fresh fruits are also a good source of fiber, which can help relieve symptoms of constipation.
- Kiwi fruit has more of vitamins C and E per serving than any other fruit. It's also a natural laxative.
- Be careful about adding alfalfa sprouts to foods you eat. Recent research has found these sprouts may increase the risk of salmonella infections in people with a weakened immune system.
- Talk to your produce grocer if you have any questions. These professionals are knowledgeable about many fruits and vegetables. They often have literature available that you can take with you.
- Fruits and vegetables you may choose from, and their serving sizes, include:
  - ~ ¾ cup vegetable juice

- ~ ½ cup broccoli, carrots or other vegetable, cooked or raw
- ~ 1 medium baked potato
- ~ 1 cup raw, leafy vegetables (greens)
- ~ ¾ cup grapes
- ~ ½ cup fruit juice
- ~ 1 medium banana, orange or apple
- ~ ¼ cup dried fruit
- ~ ¼ cup canned or cooked fruit

I don't like vegetables very much. Is it OK if I only eat fruit?

It would be better if you ate a variety of both fruits *and* vegetables. Vegetables can provide you with some nutrients not plentiful in fruits, such as the iron in dark leafy lettuce and other vegetables. Combine fruit and vegetables for a tasty serving. For example, a salad of fresh strawberries, uncooked spinach and toasted pecans served with a poppy-seed dressing provides lots of different nutrients. And it tastes great, too!

Breads, Cereal, Pasta and Rice

Carbohydrate foods provide the primary source of energy for your developing baby. These foods also ensure that your body uses protein efficiently. You need at least 6 servings from the carbohydrate group each day. Try to eat more.

- Foods from this group are nearly interchangeable, so it shouldn't be hard to get all the carbohydrates you need.
- If you don't like pasta, choose rice. If cereal isn't appealing, choose bread.
- Complex carbohydrates, such as whole-wheat breads, pastas and cereals, can be high in fiber. These are good choices because they provide your body with a constant source of energy and help you feel full longer.
- Many bread and cereal products are now fortified with folic acid. Read labels.
- Simple carbohydrates are usually full of sugar and include cookies, cake, pie and candy. Avoid eating a lot of these because they don't provide much nutrition.
- Check out what a serving size is for carbohydrates. It's easy to get more than one serving in a portion.
- Foods you might choose from this group, and their serving sizes, include:
  - ~ 1 10-inch tortilla, corn or flour
  - ~ ½ cup cooked pasta, cereal or rice
  - ~ 1 ounce ready-to-eat cereal
  - ~ ½ medium bagel
  - ~ 1 slice bread
  - ~ 1 medium roll

How many grams of carbohydrate should I eat daily during pregnancy?

There is no recommended dietary allowance (RDA) for carbohydrate intake during pregnancy. Most physicians believe carbohydrates should make up about 60% of the total number of calories in your diet. If you are eating 2200 calories a day, you would consume about 1320 calories as carbohydrate calories.

Fats and Sweets

Be careful with fats and sweets, unless you are underweight and need to add a few pounds. Foods in the fat-and-sweets group are often high in calories but low in nutritional value.

- The total of fat you consume *also* includes fats in the foods you eat, such as peanut butter, meats, milk, cheese and other foods you choose.
- Eating too many sweets during pregnancy can add weight to you *and* deprive you and baby of the nutrients you both need.
- To help control a sweet tooth, limit yourself to 100 calories of candy a day—a handful of jelly beans, four Hershey's Kisses or half a regular candy bar. Read labels!

- Be careful with your intake of butter, margarine, oils, salad dressing, nuts, chocolate and sweets.
- Replace sweet treats with nourishing choices to satisfy hunger and your nutritional needs at the same time.
- Use fats and sweets sparingly in any foods you prepare.
- In many cases, you can decrease the amount of sugar in a recipe, and it will still taste OK.
- Foods from this group, and their serving sizes, include:
  - ~ 1 tablespoon sugar or honey
  - ~ 1 tablespoon olive oil or other type of oil
  - ~ 1 pat of margarine or butter
  - ~ 1 tablespoon jelly or jam
  - ~ 1 tablespoon prepared salad dressing

I have a hard time avoiding foods that are high in sugar and fat. What can I do?

Cookies, chocolate, cake, pie, candy and ice cream have a lot of empty calories. You may have to make an effort to choose instead foods that are high in fiber and low in sugar and fat, such as fruits and vegetables, legumes and whole-grain crackers and breads. Instead of selecting a food with little nutritional value, choose a piece of fruit and some cheese or a slice of whole-wheat bread with a little peanut butter. You'll satisfy your hunger and your nutritional needs at the same time!

Facts about Fish

- Eating fish is healthy; it's particularly good for you during pregnancy.
- Experts recommend a pregnant woman eat no more than *12 ounces* of cooked fish a week; a typical fish serving is 3 to 6 ounces.
- Many fish choices are an excellent, healthful addition to your diet. They are safe to eat; you can eat them as often as you like, as long as you don't exceed 12 ounces a week.
- If you eat more than 12 ounces in one week, cut back the next week. You want to *average* 12 ounces a week.
- Fish contains omega-3 fatty acids, which help prevent some heart problems. See the discussion of omega-3 fatty acids on page 22.
- Research shows that women who eat a variety of fish during pregnancy have longer pregnancies and give birth to babies that weigh more.
- If you eat fish, you may also have fewer problems with premature labor.
- Most fish is low in fat and high in vitamin B, iron, zinc, selenium and copper.
- It's healthy to choose a variety of fish to eat.
- If you need to watch your calories, have your choices baked, broiled or steamed. Avoid lots of butter and deep frying.

- The list below contains acceptable types of fish and shellfish to choose from. (See the list of fish to avoid that begins on page 24.)

  bass (avoid large-mouth or sea bass)
  catfish, farm-raised
  clams
  crab
  croaker
  fish sticks
  flounder
  haddock
  herring
  lobster
  mackerel (avoid king mackerel)
  ocean perch
  orange roughy
  oysters (avoid Gulf Coast; limit intake of Eastern oysters)
  Pacific halibut
  perch
  perch, freshwater
  red snapper
  salmon (limit Great Lakes salmon)
  scallops
  scrod
  shrimp
  sole
  trout, farm-raised

- The FDA recommends removing the skin and as much fat as possible before you eat any type of fish.
- We advise pregnant women not to eat sushi; however, there are a couple of "sushi" dishes that are OK to eat. Sushi made with *cooked* eel and rolls with *steamed* crab and veggies are acceptable.
- Pregnant women and nursing moms should not eat some types of fish. The warning also applies to women who are planning on becoming pregnant. See the discussion that begins on page 24.

Omega-3 Fatty Acids

- Omega-3 fatty acids are oils that are good for you and your baby.
- Studies show that during pregnancy, omega-3 fatty acids may help prevent high blood pressure and pre-eclampsia.
- The omega-3 fatty acids contained in fish may also help protect you from premature labor.
- Studies have shown that fish oil is important to fetal brain development. One study showed that when a pregnant woman eats fish oil, it reaches the baby's brain.
- Anchovies, herring, mullet, mackerel (not king mackerel), salmon, sardines and trout are some fish with a lot of omega-3 fatty acids.
- Some researchers believe eating fatty fish or ingesting omega-3 fatty acids in another form (such as fish-oil capsules) may also enhance your baby's intellectual development.
- If you're a vegetarian or you don't like fish, add canola oil, flaxseed, soybeans, walnuts and wheat germ to your food plan. These foods contain linolenic oil, which is a type of omega-3 fatty acid.
- Studies show it's best not to take in more than 2.4g of omega-3 fatty acids a day.

Methyl-Mercury Poisoning and Other Poisons

- Some fish are contaminated with a dangerous substance as the result of man-made pollution.
- People who eat these fish are at risk of methyl-mercury poisoning.
- Mercury is a naturally occurring substance as well as a pollution by-product.
- It becomes a problem when it is released into the air as a pollutant. It settles into the oceans and from there winds up in some types of fish.
- The FDA has determined that a certain level of methyl mercury in fish is dangerous for humans.
- We know methyl mercury can pass from mother to fetus across the placenta.
- Because of rapid brain development, a fetus may be more vulnerable to methyl-mercury poisoning.
- Research has shown that 60,000 children are born each year who are at risk of developing neurological problems linked to the consumption of seafood by their mothers during pregnancy.
- For more information on mercury in seafood, call the FDA's toll-free hotline (1-888-SAFEFOOD) or visit its website (*vm.cfsan.fda.gov/~dms/admehg3.html*).
- Other environmental pollutants can appear in fish. Dioxin and PCBs (polychlorinated biphenyls) are

found in some fish, such as bluefish or lake trout; avoid them.

- Parasites, bacteria, viruses and toxins can also contaminate fish.
- Eating infected fish can make you sick, sometimes severely so. Sushi and ceviche are fish dishes that could contain viruses or parasites.
- Raw shellfish, if contaminated, could cause hepatitis-A, cholera or gastroenteritis.

Precautions about Fish

- **Avoid *all* raw fish during pregnancy!**
- *Do not eat* Gulf Coast oysters, halibut, king mackerel, large-mouth bass, marlin, pike, sea bass, bluefish, lake trout, shark, swordfish, tilefish, tuna steaks or tuna sushi, walleye or white croaker during your pregnancy.
- Avoid some fish found in warm tropical waters, especially Florida, the Caribbean and Hawaii. Don't eat the following "local" fish from those areas—amberjack, barracuda, grouper, mahi-mahi and snapper.
- Some freshwater fish may also be risky to eat. To be on the safe side, consult local or state authorities for any advisories on eating freshwater fish.
- Some kinds of fish should not be eaten more than once a month. These fish include blue mussels, cod,

Eastern oysters, Great Lakes salmon, Gulf of Mexico blue crab, lake whitefish, pollock and wild channel catfish.

- If you're nursing, limit your consumption of the fish listed above to once a week. Canned tuna is a little safer but don't eat more than one 6-ounce can a week.
- If you are unsure about whether you should eat a particular fish or if you would like further information, call the Food and Drug Administration on its toll-free telephone hotline: 1-800-332-4010.

I've never liked fish much, but now I seem to want to eat it all the time. Is it good for me and my baby?

Eating fish is very important during your pregnancy. It supplies vital nutrients, including omega-3 fatty acids. You should eat some fish, but don't eat more than 12 ounces in any given week. Read the list of good fish to eat, page 21, and the discussion of fish to avoid that begins on page 24. Enjoy your fish grilled, broiled or baked for a nutritious addition to your meal plan.

Vitamins and Minerals

Vitamins and minerals are an important part of your good nutrition. Pregnancy increases your need for vitamins and minerals. It's probably best if you can meet most of these needs through the foods you eat, but this may be difficult for some women. That's one reason your doctor prescribes a prenatal vitamin for you—to help you meet your increased pregnancy needs.

- For women who need extra help during pregnancy, supplements are often prescribed. These pregnant women include teenagers (whose bodies are still growing), severely underweight women, women who ate a very poor diet before conception, and women who are expecting more than one baby and who have previously given birth to multiples.
- Women who smoke or drink heavily may also need supplements.
- Pregnant women with a chronic medical condition, those who take some medications and those who have problems digesting cow's milk, wheat and other essential foods may need supplements.
- Vegetarians may need to pay special attention to their nutrition so they get enough of some essential vitamins and minerals.
- Your doctor will talk to you about vitamins and minerals. If you need more than a prenatal vitamin, he or she can give you advice.
- *Caution:* Never take any supplements without your doctor's knowledge, approval and consent!

Getting Enough Calcium

Calcium is important in the diet of every woman. The daily requirement for a nonpregnant woman is between 800 and 1000mg of calcium. When you're pregnant, your needs increase because your growing baby needs calcium to build strong bones and teeth, and you need calcium to keep your bones healthy.

- During pregnancy, your need for calcium increases to 1200mg a day.
- Your body cannot process more than 500mg of calcium at one time. Don't eat all your calcium foods at the same time.
- Most prenatal vitamins contain only a portion of the calcium you need.
- If you don't get enough calcium, your baby may draw needed calcium from your bones, which increases your risk of developing osteoporosis later in life.
- Dairy products are great sources of calcium and vitamin D, which is necessary for calcium absorption.
- It may be difficult for you to get enough calcium without eating dairy foods.
- Some foods are now calcium fortified, such as some orange juice and some breads.
- To add calcium to your diet, drink fortified juices, and eat tofu and soy milk with added calcium.

- Other nondairy foods that contain calcium include broccoli, bok choy, collards, kale, mustard greens, spinach, salmon, sardines, garbanzo beans (chickpeas), sesame seeds, almonds, dry beans and trout.
- Read nutrition labels.
- Some foods interfere with your body's absorption of calcium. Be very careful about consuming salt, protein, tea, coffee and unleavened bread with a calcium-containing food.
- If you and your doctor decide calcium supplements are necessary, you will probably be advised to take calcium carbonate combined with magnesium, which aids calcium absorption.
- Avoid any supplement derived from animal bones, dolomite or oyster shells because they may contain lead.

Lactose Intolerance

- If you are lactose intolerant, you may be able to eat hard cheeses and yogurt.
- Lactose-reduced dairy products are also available.
- Try to eat calcium-rich nondairy foods, such as figs, collard greens and fish with bones, such as sardines and anchovies.
- You may also have to take calcium supplements; discuss it with your doctor.

- You may be able to use Lactaid, a preparation that helps your body deal more efficiently with lactic acid. Ask your doctor about it.

Smart Calcium Choices
- If you need to watch your calories and avoid unnecessary fats, choose your calcium sources wisely.
- Select lowfat products and those with reduced-fat content. Skim milk and lowfat, fatfree and part-skim cheeses are better choices than whole milk and regular cheese.

Super Smoothie

By adding a few ingredients to the basic smoothie recipe, you can make this a minimeal!

½ cup skim milk or soy milk
½ cup plain lowfat or fatfree yogurt
1 medium banana
½ cup frozen fruit
2 tablespoons wheat germ
Blend all ingredients in blender until smooth. Makes one serving.

Adding Calcium to Your Meal Plan
A lot of pregnant women get tired of drinking milk or eating cheese and yogurt to meet their calcium needs during

pregnancy. Below are some suggestions of other ways to add calcium to your diet.

- Make fruit shakes with milk and fresh fruit; add a scoop of ice milk, frozen yogurt or ice cream.
- Add nonfat dried-milk powder to recipes, such as soups, mashed potatoes and meat loaf.
- Cook brown rice or oatmeal in lowfat or nonfat milk instead of water.
- Drink calcium-fortified orange juice.
- Make soups and sauces with undiluted evaporated nonfat milk instead of cream.
- Eat calcium-fortified breads.
- It may be a little difficult for you to determine how much calcium you're getting from the foods you eat.
- Package labeling usually lists the *percentage* of calcium contained in a food. This may be confusing because it's hard to know how much that is.
- The solution is to understand that labeling is based on the FDA's recommendation for a nonpregnant woman, which is 800mg a day. If a package states "calcium 20%," just multiply 800 times 0.2 (20%), which gives you the amount of 160mg.
- Keep a written record of how much calcium you get from each calcium-containing food you eat. Remember, you need 1200mg of calcium a day.

Your Folic-Acid Intake

- Folic acid (a term used interchangeably with *folate* and *vitamin B₉*) is a B vitamin that can contribute to a healthy pregnancy.

- If a mother-to-be takes 0.4mg (400 micrograms) of folic acid each day, beginning 3 or 4 months *before* pregnancy begins, it may help prevent or decrease the incidence of neural-tube defects, which are defective closures of the neural tube during early pregnancy.

- Studies have shown that about 75% of all cases can be prevented if women take folic acid before pregnancy.

- One neural-tube birth defect, called *spina bifida,* afflicts nearly 4000 babies born in the U.S. every year. It develops in the first few weeks of pregnancy.

- If a woman gives birth to a baby with spina bifida, she may need extra folic acid in later pregnancies to reduce her chances of having another baby with the same problem.

- A pregnant woman's body excretes four or five times the normal amount of folic acid.

- Folic acid is not stored in the body for very long, so it must be replaced every day.

- It's important to take in adequate amounts of folic acid, especially in your 1st trimester of pregnancy.

- Prenatal vitamins have 0.8mg to 1mg of folic acid in each pill, enough for a normal pregnancy. Most women do not need extra folic acid during pregnancy.
- Some women may need folic acid in addition to prenatal vitamins.
- Deficiency in folic acid can result in a type of anemia called *megaloblastic anemia.*
- Additional folate may be necessary for situations in which pregnancy requirements are unusually high, such as a pregnancy with twins or triplets, alcoholism or Crohn's disease.
- A folic-acid deficiency may result in anemia in you.
- Fewer than 35% of women in the U.S. of childbearing age take enough folic acid to help reduce the possibility of neural-tube defects.
- Some researchers now recommend that *all* women of childbearing age take 0.4mg of folic acid a day, in hopes of significantly decreasing the chances of this serious problem occurring.
- In 1998, the U.S. government ordered that some grain products, such as flour, breakfast cereals and pasta, be fortified with folic acid.
- Studies have shown that neural-tube defects have fallen nearly 20% since grain and cereal products began to be fortified with folic acid in 1998.

- This is important information because about 50% of all pregnancies in the U.S. are unplanned!
- Folic acid is found in many other foods, too.
- Foods that contain folic acid include asparagus, avocados, bananas, black beans, broccoli, egg yolks, fortified breads and cereals, green beans, leafy green vegetables, lentils, liver, oranges and other citrus fruits and juices, peas, plantains, spinach, strawberries, tuna, wheat germ and yogurt.
- A varied diet can help you reach your folic-acid intake goal.
- Getting enough folic acid is usually not a problem for vegetarians. Folic acid is found in many fruits, legumes and vegetables (especially dark leafy ones).
- Eating a breakfast of 1 cup of fortified cereal, with milk, and drinking a glass of orange juice supplies about half of your daily requirement of folic acid.

Fuzzy Peaches

4 ounces of chilled peach nectar
4 ounces nonalcoholic sparkling wine
dash of grenadine
Mix ingredients together in tall glass. Add ice cubes, and garnish with maraschino cherries.

Your Iron Intake

- Iron is one of the most important elements for your body; women need more iron than men because of menstruation.
- Most women do not get enough iron in their diet. Research has shown that between the ages of 20 and 50, American women consume only about 65% (10mg/day) of the Recommended Daily Allowance (RDA) of iron (15mg/day).
- The average woman's diet seldom contains enough iron to meet the increased demands of pregnancy (30mg/day).
- It's very important to meet your increased iron needs during pregnancy.
- Needs increase because your blood volume increases by 50% to support the oxygen needs of your baby and the placenta.
- However, only 10 to 15% of the iron you consume is absorbed by your body.
- Prenatal vitamins contain about 60mg of iron.
- The best type of iron to take in is "heme" iron, which comes from sources that contain blood, such as meat, poultry, eggs and fish.
- With iron that is not heme-based, the absorption rate is only about 10% and is affected by every-

thing you eat. The iron in supplements is *not* heme-based.

- So instead of taking iron supplements, you might want to try to take in heme iron to meet your iron needs.

- In the 3rd trimester, your need for iron increases even more. Your baby draws on your stores to create its own stores for the first few months of its life.

- You will also need adequate iron reserves to draw on during your baby's birth because you will lose some blood during a normal delivery.

- Researchers now believe fetuses that don't get enough iron before birth may score lower than normal on various mental and physical tests when they are older.

- If you have an iron deficiency, you may feel tired, have trouble concentrating, get sick easily or suffer from headaches, dizziness or indigestion.

- An easy way to check for iron deficiency is to examine the inside of your bottom eyelid—it should be dark pink.

- Or look at your nail beds; if you're getting enough iron, they will be pink.

- To ensure you have enough iron in your diet, eat a lot of iron-rich foods. These include chicken, lean red meat, dried fruits, organ meats, such as liver, heart and kidneys, egg yolks, spinach, kale and tofu.

- Your body stores iron efficiently, so you don't need to eat these foods every day. However, you do need to eat them on a regular basis.
- Eat vitamin-C foods and iron-rich foods together because iron is more easily absorbed by the body when consumed with vitamin C. (A spinach salad with orange sections is a nutritious example.)
- You may not need extra iron if you eat a healthful diet and take your prenatal vitamins every day. Talk to your doctor about it.
- Any iron supplements you take can cause constipation. Work with your doctor to minimize this side effect while making sure you get enough of this important mineral.
- Vegetarians and others who eat very little meat are at greater risk of iron deficiency during pregnancy.
- If you're a vegetarian, pay close attention to your iron intake. Tofu is an excellent source of iron. Most legumes and peas also contain significant amounts of the mineral. Many breakfast foods and breads are now iron fortified.
- If you are a lacto or ovo-lacto vegetarian, don't drink milk with foods that are iron rich; calcium reduces iron absorption.

- Dried fruit and dark leafy vegetables are good sources of iron.
- Cook in cast-iron pans because traces of iron will attach to whatever you're cooking.
- Some other ways to add iron to your diet include the following ideas. Try some of them.
  - ~ Add clams to your diet. Mix them in marinara sauce, or heat some clam broth, add parsley, garlic and clams, then serve over pasta.
  - ~ Instead of junk food when you want a snack, eat trail mix made of raisins, fortified cereal and nuts.
  - ~ Add molasses to cookie, bread and pancake recipes—molasses is high in iron and calcium.
- Don't drink tea or coffee with meals because tannins present in those beverages inhibit iron absorption by 75%.
- Don't take calcium and iron supplements at the same time, for better absorption of both.

Fruit Smoothie

For a cool treat!

¹⁄₂ cup frozen fruit
1 cup lowfat or fatfree flavored yogurt
¹⁄₂ cup calcium-fortified orange juice
Blend all ingredients in blender until smooth. Makes one serving.

Zinc

- Zinc stabilizes the genetic code in cells and ensures normal tissue growth in the fetus.
- It helps prevent miscarriage and premature delivery and can help regulate blood sugar in you and your baby.
- Some thin women can increase their chances of giving birth to bigger, healthier babies by taking zinc supplements during pregnancy. In one study, babies born to thin women who took zinc during pregnancy were an average 4½ ounces heavier, and head circumference was 0.16 inch larger.
- Zinc also plays a critical role in immune functions.
- In addition, zinc may help prevent stretch marks.
- Prenatal vitamins include 15 to 25mg of zinc, an adequate amount for most women.
- This mineral is found in many foods, including seafood, meat, nuts and milk.
- If you're a vegetarian, you're more likely to have a zinc deficiency, so pay close attention to getting enough zinc every day.
- Lima beans, whole-grain products, nuts, dried beans, dried peas, wheat germ and dark leafy vegetables are all good nonmeat sources of this mineral.

Vitamin A

- Vitamin A is essential to human reproduction.
- Deficiency of vitamin A in North America is rare; most women have adequate stores of the vitamin in the liver.
- What concerns doctors now is the *excessive use* of vitamin A before conception and during early pregnancy. (This concern extends only to vitamin A derived from fish oils. Vitamin A from plants is believed to be safe.)
- Studies indicate that high levels during pregnancy of vitamin A from fish oil may cause birth defects, including cleft palate and "water on the brain" (hydrocephalus).
- The RDA of vitamin A is 2700IU (international units) a day for a woman of childbearing age (5000IU is a maximum dosage).
- The requirement is the same for pregnant and non-pregnant women.
- Most women get the vitamin A they need during pregnancy from the foods they eat.
- Supplementation during pregnancy is not recommended.
- Be cautious about taking *any* substances that you have not discussed with your doctor, including vitamin A.
- If you have questions, ask your physician.

Vitamin B

- The B vitamins—B_6, B_{12} and folic acid (B_9)—influence development of nerves and red blood cells in the baby.
- Nearly 40% of all Americans are close to a deficiency in vitamin B_{12}.
- If your vitamin-B_{12} level is low, you could develop anemia during pregnancy.
- Milk, eggs, tempeh and miso provide vitamins B_6 and B_{12}. See page 31 for information on folic acid.
- Other good sources of B_6 include bananas, potatoes, collard greens, avocados and brown rice.

Vitamin E

- Vitamin E is important during pregnancy because it helps metabolize fats and helps build baby's muscles and red-blood cells.
- You can usually get enough of this vitamin if you eat meat.
- If you don't eat meat, it can be harder to get vitamin E from the rest of your diet.
- If you're a vegetarian, pay particular attention to getting enough vitamin E to meet your minimum requirements.

- Unbleached, cold-pressed vegetable oils (such as olive oil), wheat germ, spinach and dried fruits are all good sources of vitamin E.
- Read the label on your prenatal vitamin, or ask your doctor if your prenatal vitamin contains 100% of the RDA for vitamin E.
- You may want to discuss with your doctor your vitamin E intake, especially if you are a vegetarian.

Other Supplements

- The benefit of *fluoride supplementation* during pregnancy is controversial.
- Some researchers believe fluoride supplementation in a pregnant woman results in improved teeth in her child, but not everyone agrees.
- Fluoride supplementation during pregnancy has not been found to harm the baby.
- Some prenatal vitamins contain fluoride.
- You might want to talk to your doctor about taking extra *magnesium*.
- Magnesium helps to relax muscles; the uterus is a muscle.
- It might help reduce preterm labor if you take magnesium throughout your pregnancy. Ask your doctor about it.

Your Prenatal Vitamins Are Important

Did the doctor prescribe prenatal vitamins for you to take during pregnancy? Most pregnant women take a daily prenatal vitamin to meet the increased demands on their body for more vitamins and minerals while baby is growing and developing. Each prenatal vitamin contains many essential ingredients for the development of your baby and for your good health.

You should take a prenatal vitamin *every day* until your baby is born. To help you remember to take your prenatal vitamin, take it at the same time each day. For some women, taking it in the evening before bed is easier on their stomach.

Try to take your prenatal vitamin every day if you have morning sickness. Take it when you don't feel nauseous and when you're not vomiting. If you are ill, such as with the flu, and cannot keep food or liquid down, don't take your prenatal vitamin. Begin taking it again when you feel better. If you have any questions or concerns, call your doctor.

A typical prenatal vitamin contains:
- calcium to build baby's teeth and bones, and to help strengthen your own
- copper to help prevent anemia and to help bone formation
- folic acid to reduce the risk of neural-tube defects and to help blood-cell production
- iodine to help control metabolism
- iron to prevent anemia, and to help baby's blood development
- vitamin A for general health and body metabolism
- vitamin B_1 for general health and body metabolism

(continued on next page)

(continued from previous page)

- vitamin B_2 for general health and body metabolism
- vitamin B_3 for general health and body metabolism
- vitamin B_6 for general health and body metabolism
- vitamin B_{12} to promote formation of blood
- vitamin C to aid your body's absorption of iron
- vitamin D to strengthen baby's bones and teeth, and to help your body use phosphorus and calcium
- vitamin E for general health and body metabolism
- zinc to help balance fluids in your body and to aid nerve and muscle function

Drink Enough Fluids!

Water is essential to a healthy pregnancy. It enables your body to process nutrients, develop new cells, keep up with blood-volume increases and regulate body temperature.

- Your blood volume increases during pregnancy; drinking extra fluids helps you keep up with this change.
- Studies show that most people—women *and* men—do not drink enough fluid to meet their body's needs.
- You may feel better during pregnancy if you drink more liquid than you normally do.

- Research has shown that for every 15 calories you burn, your body needs about 1 tablespoon of water.
- If you burn 2000 calories a day, you need 133 tablespoons—2 quarts—of water!
- Because you need more calories during pregnancy, you also need more water.
- By the time your mouth feels parched, you have probably lost at least 2 cups of your total body water.
- Thirst is *not* a good indication of how much water you need. By the time you get thirsty, you've already lost 1% of your body's water. Don't let yourself become thirsty!
- Drink eight 8-ounce glasses (2 quarts) or more of liquid every day.
- Some women wonder if they can drink other beverages besides water. Water is the best source of fluid; however, other fluid sources help meet your needs.
- Foods and drinks that can help you get enough fluid include milk and milk products, meats, grain products, some herbal teas, fruits and juices.
- Avoid coffee, tea and diet cola as fluid sources—they can contain sodium and caffeine, which act as diuretics.
- Two quarts a day may seem like a lot of liquid to consume, but you can do it.

- Some women drink water, one glass at a time, throughout the day. (Decrease your intake later in the day so you don't have to go to the bathroom all night long.)
- Many pregnant women who suffer from headaches, uterine cramping and other problems find if they increase their fluid intake, some symptoms are relieved.
- In addition, extra fluid may provide other benefits, including boosting endurance and easing constipation.
- Drinking plenty of water also helps avoid bladder infections.
- Water is important in regulating body temperature. In fact, for each degree above 98.6F, drink an extra pint (16 ounces) of water (or other fluid) each day to help bring down a fever.
- To determine if you're drinking enough fluid, check your urine. When it is light yellow to clear, you're getting enough water. Dark-yellow urine is a sign you need to increase your fluid intake.
- When you exercise, drink a cup of water before you begin your routine. Then drink ½ cup to 1 cup of water every 20 minutes while you are exercising to help prevent dehydration.
- You might also think about drinking cranberry juice every day. A couple of glasses can help you get the

fluid you need, and it may help prevent UTIs (urinary-tract infections), especially if you were prone to them before pregnancy.
- Don't get dehydrated. Warning signs of dehydration include thirst, fatigue, weakness, dizziness and intolerance to cold.
- You can drink tap water or bottled water.
- If you choose bottled water, be sure it meets safety guidelines.
- Just because it comes from a bottle does *not* make it better.
- Water from a municipal water supply must meet minimum government safety standards, so it may be safer than bottled water in some cases.
- If your water comes from a well on your property, discuss it at one of your prenatal visits. Your doctor may have some guidelines for consuming well water.

My doctor told me to drink lots of water every day, but I hate it. Do I really need it?

Yes, you do. Extra fluid is necessary to keep up with your increased blood volume during pregnancy. You may also feel better if you drink more fluid than you normally do. Drink 6 to 8 glasses (64 ounces; 2 quarts) of fluid every day. Water is the best liquid to choose. When your urine is light yellow to clear, you're getting enough water.

Dark-yellow urine is a sign that you need to add more fluid to your diet.

Nontequila Sunrise

4 ounces cranberry juice
4 ounces pineapple juice
Mix ingredients together in a tall glass. Add ice cubes, and garnish with strawberries.

Salt, Sodium and Pregnancy

Sodium is a chemical the body needs to maintain the proper amount of fluid. Table salt is made up of sodium and chloride; about half is sodium. Too much or too little sodium can cause problems. You need some sodium; you just don't need a lot.

- During pregnancy, sodium can also affect your baby's system.
- Try to keep your consumption of sodium under 3g (3000mg) a day.
- Taking in too much sodium can cause fluid retention, swelling, bloating and problems with high blood pressure.
- You can't avoid something unless you know where to find it. With sodium, that can be tricky.

- It's in the salt shaker and in salty-tasting foods, such as pretzels, chips and salted nuts.
- It's frequently used as a preservative in foods that don't taste salty, such as canned and processed products, fast foods, cereals, desserts—even some medications.
- Read labels to see if it's in products you use, and if it is, how much a product contains.
- You can also buy inexpensive pamphlets at supermarkets and bookstores that list the sodium content of many foods, including fast foods.
- Look at the chart on page 49; it lists some foods and their sodium content.
- You can see from the lists that sodium-containing foods don't always taste salty.
- Read labels, and check other available information *before* you eat!

I've heard I should avoid sodium during pregnancy. What is it?

Sodium is a chemical that works to maintain the fluid balance in your body. You don't need to avoid all sodium—your body needs some for your metabolism to work properly. However, you don't need too much of it. During pregnancy, keep your consumption of sodium under 3g (3000mg) a day. Talk to your doctor if you take in a lot more than this or if you have problems with swelling. He or she will advise you.

Sodium Content of Some Foods

Fresh or Minimally Prepared Foods	*Amount of Sodium*
1 cup apple juice	2mg
3 apricots (fresh)	1mg
1 medium banana	1mg
1 head Boston lettuce	15mg
1 medium carrot	35mg
1 large egg	70mg
1 cup green beans (frozen)	2mg
3 ounces ground beef	60mg
1 lemon	1mg
1 cup whole milk	120mg
1 cup oatmeal (long-cooked)	10mg
1 cup orange juice	2mg
1 peach	1mg
3 ounces pork	65mg
Prepared Foods	
3 ounces bacon	1400mg
1 cup baked beans	100mg
1 slice white bread	100mg
1 frozen chicken dinner	1400mg
1 cup chicken-noodle soup	1050mg
1 cinnamon roll	630mg

(continued on next page)

(continued from previous page)

1 tablespoon cooking oil	0mg
3 ounces corned beef	1500mg
1 cup corn flakes	305mg
1 cup green beans (canned)	320mg
1 cup self-rising flour	1565mg
1 tablespoon Italian dressing	250mg
1 tablespoon catsup	155mg
1 olive	165mg
1 dill pickle	1930mg
1 cup pudding, instant	335mg
1 cup puffed rice	1mg
1 cup tomato juice	640mg

Fast Foods

1 Arby's turkey sandwich	1060mg
1 Burger King Whopper	675mg
1 Dairy Queen hot dog	990mg
1 KFC dinner (3 pieces of chicken)	2285mg
1 Taco Bell enchirito	1175mg
1 McDonald's Big Mac	1010mg

Herbal Teas and Herbs

Herbal Teas

Some types of herbal tea are good for you and help relieve certain pregnancy discomforts. Indeed, herbal tea can be a good alternative to coffee or regular tea.

"Good" Herbal Tea	Benefits
chamomile	aids digestion (avoid if you are allergic to ragweed or chrysanthemum; chamomile is in the same family)
dandelion	helps with swelling and can help soothe an upset stomach
ginger root	helps with nausea and nasal congestion
nettle leaf	rich in iron, calcium and other vitamins and minerals that you need
peppermint	relieves gas pains and calms the stomach (make this a *weak* brew; too strong and it may cause uterine contractions)
red raspberry	helps with nausea and stabilizes hormones (don't drink too much; large amounts may cause uterine contractions)

- Herbal teas you can use safely include chamomile, dandelion, ginger root, nettle leaf, peppermint and red raspberry.
- Be careful with red raspberry tea. It can help nausea; however, large amounts may stimulate contractions.
- If you are allergic to plants in the aster family (ragweed and chrysanthemums), avoid chamomile. It's

in the aster family and may cause an allergic reaction in you.

- Peppermint tea is considered safe, as long as it is *weak*. Large amounts of peppermint can cause uterine contractions.

- Some herbs and herbal teas are *not* safe to use during pregnancy because they could harm your developing baby.

- Herbs and teas to avoid during pregnancy include blue or black cohosh, pennyroyal leaf, yarrow, goldenseal, feverfew, psillium seed, mugwort, comfrey, coltsfoot, juniper, rue, tansy, cottonroot bark, large amounts of sage, senna, cascara sagrada, buckthorn, male fern, slippery elm and squaw vine.

Use of Herbs in Pregnancy

Herbs can affect you in many ways. Some herbs are safe to use during pregnancy; others are not.

- Before you take any herb, discuss it with your doctor. He or she will advise you whether it is safe to use.

- Some herbs increase the chance of bleeding and may affect blood pressure when taken within 2 weeks of delivery.

- Be very careful with alfalfa, kava, ephedra and St. John's wort. See also the list on page 51.

I often use herbal and natural medications—up to six different ones a day. These substances are safe during pregnancy, aren't they?

Treat herbs as you would prescription or over-the-counter medications. Ask *before* you take them! Herbs can be useful, but they can also be harmful when not taken appropriately. Always check with your doctor before you take any substance.

Some Food Precautions

Your Caffeine Intake

- Caffeine is a central-nervous-system stimulant; it has no known benefits for you or your baby.
- Research shows that you may be more sensitive to caffeine during pregnancy.
- For over 20 years, the FDA (Food and Drug Administration) has recommended that pregnant women avoid caffeine.
- Some researchers believe there is an association between caffeine use and miscarriage, stillbirth and premature labor.
- Caffeine crosses the placenta to the baby.

- Effects of caffeine on you during pregnancy may include irritability, headaches, stomach upset, sleeplessness and jitters.
- Smoking may compound the stimulant effect of caffeine.
- If you use caffeine, it can affect calcium metabolism in both you and your baby.
- It may be a good idea to eliminate as much as you can from your diet. It's better for your baby, and you'll probably feel better, too.
- Caffeine is a component of many beverages and foods, including coffee, tea, cola drinks and chocolate.
- Some medications, such as cough medicines and headache preparations, also contain caffeine.
- Four cups of coffee a day (800mg of caffeine) by a pregnant woman have been associated with decreased birth weight and a smaller head size in newborns.
- An intake of 400mg a day of caffeine by a pregnant woman may affect her baby's developing respiratory system and may increase the chances of breathing problems in a newborn.
- One study showed caffeine exposure before birth might be linked to sudden infant death syndrome (SIDS).

- An exact "toxic" amount for caffeine has not been determined, but it makes sense to limit your intake.
- Read labels on foods, beverages and over-the-counter medications to determine caffeine content. Eliminate as much caffeine from your diet as possible.
- If you're jittery, your baby may suffer from the same effects.
- Caffeine passes to breast milk, which may cause irritability and sleeplessness in a breastfed baby. An infant metabolizes caffeine slower than an adult, and caffeine can collect in the infant.
- Most professionals agree that up to two cups (*not mugs*) of regular coffee or its equivalent each day is probably OK. Keep your intake under 200mg a day.
- See the list below for some sources of caffeine and their amounts.
  - ~ coffee, 5 ounces—from 60 to 140mg
  - ~ tea, 5 ounces—from 30 to 65mg
  - ~ baking chocolate, 1 ounce—25mg
  - ~ chocolate candy, 1 ounce—6mg
  - ~ soft drinks, 12 ounces—from 35 to 55mg
  - ~ pain-relief tablets, standard dose—40mg
  - ~ allergy and cold remedies, standard dose—25mg

I drink a few cups of coffee and several glasses of diet cola every day. Do I need to worry about caffeine?

Although we don't know how much caffeine is too much, it makes sense to limit your caffeine intake. Drinking 4 cups of coffee a day (800mg of caffeine) during pregnancy has been associated with problems in newborns. Eliminate caffeine from your diet, or use as little as possible.

Sweet Lemon Tea

A refreshing lift.

6 cups unsweetened decaffeinated tea
$^3/_4$ cup sugar or equivalent amount of Splenda
$^1/_3$ cup lemon juice
Combine tea, sugar or sugar substitute and lemon juice in large pitcher. Chill. Makes 7 cups.

Listeriosis

Some foods made from milk and foods from other sources should be avoided by a pregnant woman. These foods include unpasteurized milk, any food made from unpasteurized milk, soft cheeses such as Brie, Camembert, feta, goat, queso fresco and Roquefort, deli meats, undercooked poultry, undercooked meat, undercooked seafood and undercooked hot dogs. They are a common source of a form of food poisoning called *listeriosis.*

- Listeriosis can be serious for a pregnant woman and her growing baby.
- It can cause miscarriage and premature labor.
- Symptoms of listeriosis include muscle aches, fever, diarrhea and upset stomach. These symptoms may occur up to *1 month* after eating a contaminated food.
- Your doctor can screen for listeriosis with a simple blood test. Treatment with antibiotics can help prevent problems in baby.
- Avoiding listeriosis is not difficult if you follow the guidelines below.
- Drink only pasteurized milk and juice. Do not eat foods that contain unpasteurized milk.
- Eat only pasteurized cheese; hard cheeses, cream cheese and yogurt are safe.
- Avoid soft cheeses such as brie, Camembert, blue-veined, feta, goat and queso fresco.
- Don't eat uncooked or undercooked hot dogs. Be sure they are heated until steaming.
- Cold cuts and deli meats may be hazardous because they are often underprocessed. Heat them to steaming for safety.

- Don't eat refrigerated meat spreads and paté.
- Refrigerated smoked seafood should not be eaten; this includes any fish labeled "kippered," "smoked," "nova-style," "lox" or "jerky."
- If you are unsure about a food, especially when eating out, avoid it!

Other Food Warnings and Precautions

Peanut Allergy

- *Peanut allergy* is on the rise in the U.S.—about 1½ million Americans are already affected to some degree.
- If you or your partner have a strong family history of any type of allergies, avoid peanuts during pregnancy.
- Don't eat peanuts or peanut products if you breastfeed.
- Avoid other tree-grown nuts, including walnuts, almonds, hazelnuts, pecans and cashews.
- In addition, don't eat fish or eggs, and don't drink cow's milk. This will help avoid exposing your baby to some common allergens.
- Don't let your child have any peanuts or peanut products until age 3.

PKU

- *Phenylketonuria* (PKU) is a condition in which the body is unable to use phenylalanine properly, and it accumulates in body fluids.
- Accumulation can lead to mental retardation and other nervous-system disorders in you or your developing baby.
- If you suffer from phenylketonuria, follow a diet low in phenylalanine.
- Avoid the artificial sweetener aspartame.

Salmonella

- *Salmonella poisoning* is caused by bacteria.
- Almost 1400 strains have been identified.
- Any form of salmonella could be dangerous to a pregnant woman.
- Problems range from mild gastric distress to severe, sometimes fatal, food poisoning.
- This situation can be serious for a pregnant woman and her developing baby if it prevents her from getting enough fluid or eating nutritiously.
- Salmonella bacteria can be found in raw chicken and other raw poultry.
- Cracked raw eggs can be contaminated with salmonella organisms. These organisms can be found in

uncracked eggs as well, if a hen's ovaries are contaminated.

- Bacteria are destroyed in cooking, but it's prudent to take additional precautions against salmonella poisoning.
  - ~ After food preparation, clean counters, utensils, dishes and pans with a disinfecting agent.
  - ~ Wash your hands after preparing any poultry or products made with raw eggs. You could pick up salmonella on your hands from these surfaces and transfer it to your mouth or another surface.
  - ~ Thoroughly cook all poultry.
  - ~ Avoid foods made with raw eggs, including salad dressings (Caesar salad), hollandaise sauce, eggnog, homemade ice cream made with eggs or any other food made with raw or undercooked eggs.
  - ~ Don't eat cookie dough or cake batter or anything else that contains raw eggs.
  - ~ Boil eggs at least 7 minutes for hard-cooked eggs.
  - ~ Poach eggs for 5 minutes.
  - ~ Fry eggs for 3 minutes on *each* side.
  - ~ Avoid "sunny-side up" eggs (those not turned during frying). Cook the entire egg thoroughly, not just part of it.
- Be careful about adding alfalfa sprouts to foods you eat. Recent research has found that these sprouts

may increase the risk of salmonella infections in people with a weakened immune system.

Food Additives and Pesticides

- When possible, avoid *food additives.*
- We aren't really sure how they can affect a developing baby, but if you can avoid them, do so.
- Be careful about *pesticides* on foods, too.
- Thoroughly wash and wipe dry all fruits and vegetables before you eat or prepare them. Contaminants could get on your hands if you don't.
- Even if you normally peel it before eating, wash the fruit or vegetable first. It helps remove even more of any contaminated substances.

Artificial Sweeteners

Many women use artificial sweeteners to help cut calories. In general, we suggest you don't use artificial sweeteners or food additives during pregnancy, if you can avoid them.

- It's probably best to eliminate any substance you don't really need from the foods you eat and the beverages you drink for your good and the good of your baby.
- Aspartame and saccharin are the two most common artificial sweeteners added to foods and beverages.

- *Aspartame* (sold under the brand names Nutrasweet and Equal) may be the most popular artificial sweetener. It is also used in many foods and beverages to help reduce calorie content.
- Aspartame is a combination of phenylalanine and aspartic acid, two amino acids.
- There has been controversy as to the safety of aspartame use during pregnancy.
- We advise you to substitute foods that do not contain the sweetener. At this point, we're unsure about its safety for pregnant women and their developing babies.
- If you suffer from phenylketonuria, you must follow a low-phenylalanine diet or your baby may be adversely affected. Phenylalanine in aspartame contributes to phenylalanine in the diet.
- *Saccharin* is another artificial sweetener used in many foods and beverages. Although it is not used as much today as in the past, it still appears in many foods, beverages and other substances.
- The Center for Science in the Public Interest reports that testing of saccharin does not indicate it is safe to use during pregnancy.
- It would probably be better to avoid using this product while you're pregnant.

- In 1998, the Food and Drug Administration approved the use of *Splenda* as a sweetener in a wide variety of food products.
- Splenda is a trade name for a low-calorie sweetener called *sucralose,* and it is made from sugar.
- Sucralose passes through the body without being metabolized—your body does not recognize it as either a sugar or a carbohydrate, which makes it low calorie.
- At this time, sucralose is being used in salad dressings, baked goods, desserts, dairy products, beverages, jams and jellies, coffee and tea, syrups and chewing gum.
- Splenda is safe for pregnant and nursing women to use.
- You can buy it in various forms at the grocery store. You can even cook and bake with it, just like real sugar.

When You're
Eating for More than Two

If you're expecting more than one baby, your nutrition and weight gain are extremely important during your pregnancy. See the discussion of weight gain for a multiple pregnancy beginning on page 133.

- When you are carrying more than one baby, your babies will draw more nutrients from your body than if you are carrying only one, so double your efforts to eat well.
- When you are eating for yourself and two or more babies, you face a pretty big challenge.
- It's important to gain weight in the first half of pregnancy. That way, you have stores for your babies to use later.
- If you don't gain weight early in pregnancy, you are more likely to develop pre-eclampsia.
- Your babies are also more likely to be significantly smaller at birth.
- A good goal to set is to gain 24 pounds by 24 weeks with twins and 34 pounds by 24 weeks with triplets.
- You should be eating about 3500 calories a day for twins and 4500 calories a day for triplets.
- Eating six to eight small meals a day is better for you than if you only eat three large meals.
- If you eat six times a day, aim for about 600 calories per meal if you are carrying twins and 750 calories per meal if you're carrying triplets.
- Food is your best source of nutrients and calories, but it's also important for you to take your prenatal vitamin every day.

- Taking a daily prenatal vitamin provides some assurance that you are getting some of the nutrients you need.
- Good food choices can provide you with adequate protein, calories and calcium.
- Just adding extra calories won't benefit you or your developing babies. Try to get your calories from specific sources.
- Be sure to add one more serving each of dairy products and protein each day. These two servings provide you with the extra calcium, protein and iron to meet the needs of your growing babies.
- In addition, dietary supplements can help you a great deal. Zinc is one supplement to discuss with your doctor. It helps fight infection, and it may help reduce your chances of getting stretch marks. Zinc may also help your babies gain weight.
- Magnesium helps control muscles. It may reduce your chances of preterm labor.
- You will probably need more iron, too. Try to get your extra iron from food sources such as red meat, poultry, eggs and fish. The iron from iron supplements is not used as efficiently by your body. Only about 10% of supplemental iron is absorbed by your body.
- Extra calcium is a must for you now. If your babies don't get enough calcium from your nutrition, they will take it from your bones.

- You need about 3 grams of calcium each day for the good health of your bones and the good health of your babies' bones and teeth. And extra calcium may help reduce the risk of pre-eclampsia.
- Plan your food intake carefully. Eat proteins and carbohydrates together to help stabilize your blood sugar.
- A serving from the dairy group before bed is a good idea. It helps maintain your blood sugar level during the night because it is metabolized slowly.

The Challenge of Being Vegetarian during Pregnancy

Some women choose to eat a meatless diet for personal or religious choices; other women find that during pregnancy, the sight of meat makes them sick. Many women want to know if eating a vegetarian diet—a food plan without meat—is safe during pregnancy.

- Following a vegetarian diet while you're pregnant can be safe and healthful, if you pay close attention to the foods and combinations of foods you eat.
- Most women who eliminate meat from their diets eat a more nutrient-rich variety of foods than those who eat meat.

- These women may make an extra effort to include more fruits and vegetables in their food plans when they eliminate meat products.
- If you are a vegetarian, you need to be sure you eat enough calories to fuel your pregnancy.
- During pregnancy, you need to consume between 2200 and 2700 calories a day, depending on your prepregnancy weight.
- In addition to eating enough calories, you must eat the *right* kind of calories.
- Choose fresh foods that provide a variety of vitamins and minerals.
- Avoid too many fat calories because you may gain extra weight.
- Avoid empty calories that have little or no nutritional value.
- If you have questions, be sure to discuss them with your doctor. He or she may want you to see a nutritionist if you have any pregnancy risk factors.
- If you're a vegetarian, discuss your daily diet with your doctor at your first prenatal visit.

Different Vegetarian Diets

Different vegetarian nutrition plans have unique characteristics. If you are a *lacto vegetarian,* your diet includes

Veggie-Cheese Wrap

1 10-inch fatfree flour tortilla
½ cup shredded cheese (lowfat or fatfree)
4 slices tomato
¼ avocado, peeled and sliced thin
2 tablespoons mild salsa
Place tortilla on a plate. Top with shredded cheese; microwave until cheese melts (about 15 seconds). Top with tomato slices, avocado slices and salsa. Roll and enjoy!

milk and milk products. If you are an *ovo-lacto vegetarian,* your eating plan includes milk products and eggs. A *vegan* diet includes only foods of plant origin, such as nuts, seeds, vegetables, fruits, grains and legumes. A *macrobiotic* diet limits foods to whole grains, beans, vegetables and moderate amounts of fish and fruits. A *fruitarian* diet is the most restrictive; it allows only fruits, nuts, olive oil and honey. Whatever specific kind of vegetarian you are, here are some things to keep in mind.

- Your goal is to eat enough calories to gain weight during pregnancy.
- You don't want your body to use protein for energy because you need it for your growth and your baby's growth.
- You may also need to be concerned about your mineral intake.

- By eating a wide variety of whole grains, legumes, dried fruit, lima beans and wheat germ, you should be able to get enough iron, zinc and other trace minerals.

- If you don't drink milk or include milk products in your diet, you must find other sources of vitamins D, B_2, B_{12} and calcium.

- Getting enough folic acid is usually not a problem for vegetarians. Folic acid is found in many fruits, legumes and vegetables (especially dark leafy ones).

- Vegetarians and others who eat very little meat are at greater risk of iron deficiency during pregnancy.

- To get enough iron, eat an assortment of grains, vegetables, seeds and nuts, legumes and fortified cereal every day. Spinach, prunes and sauerkraut are excellent sources of iron, as are dried fruit and dark leafy vegetables. Tofu is also an excellent source of iron.

- Cook in cast-iron pans because traces of iron will attach to whatever you're cooking.

- If you are a lacto or ovo-lacto vegetarian, do not drink milk with foods that are iron rich; calcium reduces iron absorption.

- Don't drink tea or coffee with meals because tannins present in those beverages inhibit iron absorption by 75%.

- To get omega-3 fatty acids, add canola oil, flaxseed, soybeans, walnuts and wheat germ to your food plan because these foods contain linolenic oil, which is a type of omega-3 fatty acid.

- Vegetarians and pregnant women who can't eat meat may have a harder time getting enough vitamin E.
- Vitamin E is important during pregnancy because it helps metabolize polyunsaturated fats and contributes to building muscles and red-blood cells. Foods rich in the vitamin include olive oil, wheat germ, spinach and dried fruit.
- If you are a vegetarian, you are more likely to have a zinc deficiency, so pay close attention to getting enough zinc every day. Lima beans, whole-grain products, nuts, dried beans, dried peas, wheat germ and dark leafy vegetables are all good sources of zinc.
- As an ovo-lacto vegetarian, the fact that you eat egg products and dairy products means it won't be too hard for you to eat what you need, although it may be difficult for you to get enough iron and zinc.
- As a vegan, eating no animal products may make your task more difficult.
- You may need to ask your doctor about supplements for vitamin B_{12}, vitamin D, zinc, iron and calcium.
- Adding turnip greens, spinach, beet greens, broccoli, soy-based milk products and cheeses, and fruit juices fortified with calcium to your diet may be helpful.

- Macrobiotic and fruitarian diets are too restrictive for a pregnant woman. They do not provide the vitamins, minerals, protein and calories you need for baby's development. Avoid them.

Green, Yellow and Red Veggie Bake

Get your nutrients in this yummie side dish!

Cooking spray or olive oil for sautéeing
1 large zucchini, sliced
1 to 2 yellow squashes, sliced
1 to 2 onions, cut in medium chunks
3 to 4 tomatoes, cut in medium chunks
garlic to taste

Spray bottom of large frying pan with cooking spray or pour in olive oil; heat. Add all vegetables, and stir. Cover pan and cook thoroughly, from 45 minutes to an hour. Serve as main course with rice, or serve as a side dish.

Part II: Eating Wisely throughout Your Pregnancy

Morning Sickness

You may have to deal with nausea and vomiting during pregnancy; it is also called *morning sickness*. The hormone that makes a home pregnancy test change color— HCG (human chorionic gonadotropin)—also causes morning sickness. Researchers believe the problem may also be caused by an imbalance in vitamin B_6. Not every woman has morning sickness, but many women do suffer from it. You may have morning sickness at any time of day, and it may last all day long.

- The condition usually begins around week 6 and lasts until week 12 or 13, when it starts to taper off. Unfortunately, sometimes morning sickness can last all through pregnancy.
- A pill, available by prescription, may help relieve the symptoms of morning sickness; it is called *Bendectin*.
- If you are suffering from nausea and vomiting, call your doctor's office. Ask about Bendectin, especially if your first prenatal appointment isn't for a while.

- Your body needs lots of fluid all during pregnancy, especially if you lose fluids when you vomit. If you are nauseated, try to keep drinking fluids, even if you can't eat.
- Brush your teeth with toothpaste after vomiting. Stomach acids can be very hard on teeth.
- Let your boss know you have morning sickness and that you may miss work sometimes.
- If morning sickness causes you to miss work, the Family and Medical Leave Act (FMLA) states you do *not* need a doctor's note about the problem. However, most doctors will be happy to give you a note if you want one.
- If you normally cook meals, you may want to ask your partner to do it for a while. Your sense of smell may be extra sensitive, which can make you feel sick.
- If certain foods make you ill, ask your partner not to eat them around you.
- Ask people not to talk about food if just hearing about it makes you want to throw up.
- Acupressure, acupuncture, massage and hypnosis may help you deal with nausea and vomiting.
- Don't take herbs, over-the-counter treatments or any other "remedies" for nausea that are not known to be safe during pregnancy.

Apricot Cooler

For a great change of pace.

2 cups apricot nectar
2 cups unsweetened pineapple juice
⅓ cup lemon juice
1 can ginger ale, chilled
Combine apricot nectar, pineapple juice and lemon juice in large pitcher. Chill. Just before serving, add ginger ale. Makes 6 cups.

When Nausea Is a Severe Problem

- A severe form of morning sickness is called *hyperemesis gravidarum.*
- With hyperemesis gravidarum, a woman has severe nausea, dehydration and vomiting during pregnancy.
- A woman with hyperemesis gravidarum may also need to be admitted to the hospital, usually to receive I.V.s to help with dehydration and to receive injectable medications for nausea.
- Hypnosis and/or acupuncture may help a woman deal with the problem.

Some Helpful Hints for Dealing with Morning Sickness

- Eat small meals frequently to keep your stomach from being overfull. A full stomach (or an empty one) may make you feel sick.

- Drink lots of fluids. Fluids may be easier to handle than solids, and they help you avoid dehydration. Dehydration is more serious than not eating for a while.
- If you vomit a lot, you may want to choose fluids that contain electrolytes to help replace those you lose when you vomit. Ask your doctor what fluids to drink.
- Find out what foods or smells make you sick. Avoid them when possible.
- Don't drink coffee because it produces stomach acid, which can make you feel sick.
- A high-protein snack or a high-carbohydrate snack before bed may help you feel better.
- Try some "pregnancy lollipops" to help deal with the problem. Pops are now available to help reduce nausea and dry mouth, and they come in a variety of flavors. Ask about them at your drugstore or food market.
- Ask your partner to bring you some dry toast, rice cakes or crackers in the morning for you to eat before you get up. Or keep dry cereal nearby so you can nibble on it before you get out of bed. These foods all help absorb stomach acid.
- Be sure you get enough rest.
- Keep your bedroom cool at night, and air it out often. Cool air and/or fresh air may help you feel better.
- Get out of bed slowly.

- If you take an iron supplement, take it an hour before meals or 2 hours after a meal.
- Nibble on raw ginger, or pour boiling water over it and sip the "tea." It's a natural remedy for nausea.
- Salty foods help some women feel better.
- Lemonade and watermelon may help alleviate symptoms. Cut up a fresh lemon to suck on when you feel nauseous.
- Eat what appeals to you—foods that are appealing may be the ones you can keep down more easily right now. If that means whole-wheat crackers and root beer, go for it!
- Some women find that protein foods settle more easily in the stomach; these foods include cheese, eggs, peanut butter and nonfatty meats.
- Avoid other things that make you ill, such as odors, movement or noise.
- Try a motion-sickness bracelet or wristband; it may help relieve nausea.
- A device called the *ReliefBand* uses gentle electrical signals to stimulate the nerves in the wrist; this stimulation is believed to interfere with messages between the brain and stomach that cause nausea. It is safe to use during pregnancy.
- The band has various stimulation levels that allow you to adjust signals for maximum control for your

individual comfort. It can be used when nausea begins, or you can wear it before you feel ill.
• ReliefBand does not interfere with eating or drinking. It is water resistant and shock resistant, so you can wear it just about any time!

Be Prepared When You Go Out

• When you're away from home, take along a "morning sickness" emergency traveling bag. It can come in handy, especially if you suffer from nausea and vomiting throughout the day.
• With your emergency bag along, you'll be able to handle this temporary side effect of pregnancy, no matter where you are.
• In a sturdy bag, pack along the following:
  ~ some opaque plastic bags (plastic grocery sacks are a good choice), without holes
  ~ wet wipes, tissue or napkins to wipe your face and mouth
  ~ a small bottle of water to rinse your mouth and teeth
  ~ a toothbrush and toothpaste to brush away stomach acids
  ~ a small bottle of breath spray or breath mints

Some Common Solutions to Pregnancy Problems Associated with Food

- If you have an upset stomach, eat a banana. A recent study showed bananas cause the stomach to produce mucus and other cells that help protect the lining, which may protect against irritation.

- If you experience diarrhea, add a little sugar to a cup of tea or lemon water. Sugar helps the intestines absorb water instead of passing it.

- If excessive gas is a problem, eat small amounts of food and chew every mouthful thoroughly. Avoid gas-producing foods, such as cabbage, onions and Brussels sprouts.

- If you suffer from heartburn, drink a small amount of milk about 20 minutes before your meal to help prevent the problem.

- Exercise may help prevent some forms of stomach upset.

- If you have problems with swelling, be careful with foods high in sodium. Although you may really want those potato chips or that pickle, you may pay for it later with swollen ankles or swollen fingers.

- Have a pregnancy "minimeal" for taste and nutrition, and to help you deal with some common pregnancy discomforts. See the *Super Smoothie* recipe on page 29. This super smoothie passes through the stomach quickly, to help avoid heartburn. It is absorbed into the bloodstream slowly, for good sugar balance and constant nutrient supply. It leaves the intestines quickly, to prevent constipation. And it provides calcium, fiber and protein. You can't miss with this yummy treat!

I feel so sick to my stomach that I can't eat anything. Is this dangerous?

Nausea is not usually dangerous because it doesn't last too long. It becomes dangerous when you can't eat enough food or drink enough fluid. Morning sickness is usually bad during the beginning of pregnancy. It usually gets better and disappears after the 1st trimester, then you should feel better for the rest of your pregnancy.

Cravings and Food Aversions

Food Cravings

Desire (cravings) for particular foods during pregnancy is normal for many women. Indeed, food cravings have long been considered a nonspecific sign of pregnancy.

- You may be surprised by some of the weird foods you want to eat and sometimes the food you want appears a little strange to other people!
- For years, comedians used "pickles and ice cream" as a craving many pregnant women had.
- You may find your cravings are not that strange, or they may be stranger!

- We don't know why women sometimes crave un-usual foods or unusual food combinations during pregnancy.
- Hormonal and emotional changes that occur dur-ing pregnancy may have something to do with it.
- Cravings can be both good and bad.
- If you crave foods that are nutritious and healthful, go ahead and eat them in moderate amounts.
- If you crave foods that are high in sugar and fat, loaded with empty calories, be careful about eating them.
- There are ways to help yourself when you have food cravings. Try the following, and you'll be able to in-dulge a little:
  - ~ "downsize it"—satisfy a craving by having only one or two bites
  - ~ slow down—when you eat and drink *slowly,* you give your brain a chance to realize you're satisfied
  - ~ substitute—when you crave one food, try substitut-ing something else for it (see the box on page 82)

Pica

- There is a condition in which pregnant women crave nonfood items, such as ice, clay, coffee grounds, corn starch, wax and other substances.

Can You Give In to Cravings?

"Giving in" to your cravings doesn't mean you can't do it in a healthy way. Use the following substitutions to help you get what you want.

- when you crave chocolate—try cold chocolate skim milk or hot chocolate made from skim milk
- when you crave potato chips—try lowfat bagel chips, pretzels, baked tortilla chips, seasoned rice cakes, oyster crackers, popcorn
- a sweet dessert—small bran muffin, baked yam, tapioca, toast with honey or jelly, small slice of angel food cake, frozen juice bars
- candy—a glass of lemonade or drink mix made with Splenda, a frozen banana, dried fruit, melon pieces
- something creamy—lowfat or nonfat frozen yogurt, lowfat or fatfree ice milk, smoothies, pudding, tapioca or healthy shakes

- This kind of craving is called *pica*, and it isn't healthy for you or your baby.
- If you allow yourself to eat these kinds of things, it can cause a variety of problems, including blocked bowels, nutritional deficiencies and severe constipation.
- If you have cravings for nonfood items, talk to your doctor about them.

- He or she may prescribe a supplement, usually iron, to help deal with the problem.

Food Aversions

- On the opposite side of cravings is *food aversions.*
- Some foods that you have eaten without problems before pregnancy may now make you sick to your stomach.
- This is common so don't be surprised if you can't stand the sight of some food you normally love.
- As with cravings, we believe the hormones of pregnancy are involved in aversions.
- With food aversions, hormones impact on the gastrointestinal tract, which can affect your reaction to some foods.
- If a food your partner enjoys is one that nauseates you, ask him to fix it on his own.
- Tell him you may not be able to sit with him when he eats it.
- Ask him to prepare it when you're not around or to eat it when he is out, such as at lunch, when you aren't with him.
- When he's finished, ask him to clean up his pans and dishes. Just washing up the cooking utensils may make you feel ill!

I've been craving certain foods now that I'm pregnant. Is this normal?

For many women, cravings during pregnancy are normal. Be careful about giving in to your cravings. If you desire foods that are high in sugar and fat, and loaded with empty calories, be careful about eating them. They could add unnecessary, empty calories to your food plan. If you crave nonfood items, talk with your doctor about it.

Junk Food and Snacking

Eating Junk Food

Is junk food your kind of food? Do you eat it several times a day?

- "Junk food" is high-calorie, high-fat food that contains little nutrition for you or your baby.
- Pregnancy is the time to curb the junk-food habit!
- Now that you're pregnant, your food intake affects someone besides just yourself—your growing baby.
- If you're used to skipping breakfast, getting something "from a machine" for lunch, then eating din-

ner at a fast-food restaurant, it doesn't help your pregnancy.

- You may have to forgo most junk food while you're pregnant.
- It's OK to eat some now and then, but don't make it a regular part of your diet.
- Avoid chips, sodas, cookies, pie, chocolate, candy, cake, ice cream and many fast foods. Instead, select foods that are high in fiber and low in sugar and fat; choose fruits and vegetables, legumes, dairy products and whole-grain crackers and breads.

I love junk food. Do I have to give it up completely?

You may not be able to eat much junk food during pregnancy. The foods we consider "junk" are usually foods that contain little nutrition for you or your baby, but they do contain a lot of calories. It's probably OK to eat junk food once in awhile, but don't make it a regular part of your diet.

Snacking at Night

- Late-night nutritious snacks are beneficial for some women, especially if they must eat many small meals a day.

- However, many women should not snack at night because they don't need the extra calories.
- For others, food in the stomach late at night can cause heartburn or indigestion.

Smart Snacking

You may not feel much like eating at times during your pregnancy, but it's important to keep eating a healthy diet. Snacks might be the answer.

- Instead of eating large meals, eat small snacks throughout the day to keep your energy levels up and to help avoid heartburn and indigestion.
- Pregnant women should snack often, particularly in the second half of pregnancy.
- You should have three or four snacks a day, in addition to your regular meals.
- There are a couple of catches though. First, meals may need to be smaller so you can eat those snacks. Second, snacks must be nutritious.
- What you eat and when you eat become more important when you realize how your actions affect your baby.
- If you work, take healthful foods with you for snacks and lunches; stay away from fast food and junk food.

- Smart snacks can add nutrition and taste to your eating plan.
- Below are some helpful tips.
  - ~ Know what time of day or night hunger strikes you the hardest and prepare things in advance. Cut up fresh vegetables for later use in salads and for munching with low-cal dip.
  - ~ Keep some hard-cooked eggs on hand.
  - ~ Peanut butter (reduced-fat or regular), pretzels and plain popcorn are good, quick choices.
  - ~ Fruit juice can replace soda. If juice has more sugar than you need, cut it with water.
  - ~ Some herbal teas can be good for you. See the discussion of herbal teas beginning on page 50.
  - ~ Try something different if you're bored with the foods you've been eating—guacamole on baked tortilla chips, artichoke-spinach dip on a baked potato or black-bean dip and raw veggies are some good alternatives.
  - ~ Avoid lowfat and fatfree foods made with olestra because it may deplete vital nutrients baby needs for growth. It can also cause stomach problems and excessive gassiness in you.
  - ~ When you're looking for something to snack on, you might not think of a baked potato, but it's an

excellent snack! You get protein, fiber, calcium, iron, B vitamins and vitamin C when you eat a potato. Bake up a few potatoes, and keep them in the refrigerator. Heat one up when you're hungry.

~ Broccoli is another food filled with vitamins. Add it to your baked potato, and top both with some plain yogurt or nonfat sour cream for a delicious treat!

- The list below offers some nutritious snacks. Try some of them, or use these ideas to create your own.

  ~ bananas, raisins, dried fruit and mangoes to satisfy your sweet tooth and to provide you with iron, potassium and magnesium

  ~ string cheese; it's high in calcium and protein

  ~ fruit shakes made with milk and yogurt or ice cream provide calcium, vitamins and minerals

  ~ crackers that are high in fiber; spread with a little peanut butter for added taste and some protein

  ~ cottage cheese and fruit, flavored with a little sugar or Splenda, and some cinnamon, for a tasty milk-and-fruit serving

  ~ salt-free chips or tortillas with salsa or bean dip for fiber and good taste

  ~ humus and pita slices for fiber and good taste

- ~ fresh tomatoes, flavored with some olive oil and fresh basil; eat with a few thin slices of Parmesan cheese for a dairy serving and a vegetable serving
  - ~ chicken or tuna salad (made from fresh chicken or tuna packed in water) and crackers or tortilla pieces for protein and fiber
- Snacks that contain lots of vitamins and minerals but only 100 to 150 calories include the following:
  - ~ a baked apple with nutmeg, 1 teaspoon of sugar or 1 packet of Splenda, and cinnamon
  - ~ a package of instant oatmeal
  - ~ a cup of fresh fruit
  - ~ a veggie burger on a slice of whole-wheat bread
  - ~ a cup of gelatin or pudding
  - ~ a cup of fresh veggies and 1/4 cup lowfat dip

I've found that I want to eat late at night, even though I've never felt hungry at night before. Should I eat late at night?

Late-night nutritious snacks are beneficial for some women, especially if they must eat many small meals a day. However, many women should not snack at night because they don't need the extra calories. Food in the stomach late at night may also cause more distress if heartburn or nausea and vomiting are problems.

Eating Out

Many pregnant women are concerned about eating out. Some want to know if they should avoid certain types of food, such as Mexican, Vietnamese, Thai, Indian or Greek food. As you might be, they're concerned that certain foods could be harmful to the baby.

- It's OK to eat out, just be careful about what you eat because certain foods might not agree with you.
- The best types of foods to eat at restaurants are those you tolerate well at home.
- At a restaurant, your best choices may be chicken, lean meat or fish, fresh vegetables and salads.
- Be careful with calorie-loaded salad dressings if you are concerned about excessive weight gain.
- Don't eat raw meats or raw seafood, such as sushi.
- Avoid foods that may not agree with you right now.
- Avoid restaurants that serve highly salted foods, foods high in sodium or foods loaded with calories and fat, such as gravies, fried foods, junk food and rich desserts. It may be difficult to control your calorie intake at some restaurants.
- Be careful with portions. Many restaurants serve very large portions; these can contain a lot of unnecessary calories.

- One way to control the size of your portions is to ask the waiter to box half of the food on your plate *before* he or she brings your meal to you. Or ask for a to-go box when your meal is served so you can box some of the food before you even start eating!
- Chinese food often contains large amounts of MSG (monosodium glutamate, a sodium-containing product). You may retain water after eating these foods.
- You may wonder what kinds of foods you can eat if you're out and about, in a hurry or didn't have time to make lunch.
- Many fast-food restaurants are making an effort to provide their customers with nutritious, lowfat food choices.
- If you're unsure what may be best for you, ask the manager for the nutritional guidelines for the foods the restaurant serves.
- Some places have a brochure you can take with you; some have the guidelines in books that they can let you look at while you're there. Some places have the information right on the menu!
- Nutrition information usually includes the serving size, the number of calories in a serving and the amount of fat. It may also contain other important information, such as the amount of sodium,

carbohydrates, dietary fiber, protein, vitamins A and C, calcium and iron.

- Having this information available helps you make wise choices. You may not have to give up some of the foods you love.
- You can still occasionally eat fast food—and you'll be able to make healthy choices when you do!
- Another challenge is maintaining a healthy diet if you work outside your home.
- It may be necessary to go to business lunches or to travel for your company.
- Be selective. If you can choose off the menu, look for "healthy" or lowfat choices.
- You might want to ask about preparation—instead of frying, maybe a dish can be broiled.
- On a business trip, take along some of your own food.
- Choose healthy nonperishables, such as whole-grain crackers and peanut butter or fruits and vegetables that don't need refrigeration.

Going to Parties

You and your partner have been invited to a big party. You've been very diligent about your nutrition, and you're pregnancy is almost over. Should you let yourself go, and eat and drink whatever you want?

Sweeta Margarita

3 ounces fresh or frozen mixed berries, sweetened to taste with sugar
  or Splenda, if necessary
1 ounce lime juice
2 ounces of pineapple juice
dash of sparkling water

*Place berries, lime juice and pineapple juice in shaker. Let sit for ¹/₂
  hour. Wet the rim of a margarita glass with lime juice, then dip the
  glass in sugar. Set glass aside. To the mixture in the shaker, add a
  dash of sparkling water. Using a strainer, strain the mixture from the
  shaker into the prepared margarita glass. Garnish with a spear of
  fresh berries.*

- It's probably a good idea to maintain your good eating habits.
- You *can* party healthfully.
- Below are some suggestions to keep in mind to help you have a good time.
  - ~ Eat something before you go to take the edge off your appetite. It may be easier to avoid high-fat and high-calorie foods if you're not ravenous.
  - ~ Eat food when it's fresh and/or hot—at the beginning of the party. As the party goes on, the food may not be chilled or heated enough to prevent bacteria from growing. So eat early.
  - ~ Avoid alcohol. Instead drink fruit juice "spiked" with ginger ale or lemon-lime soda.

~ If it's the holiday season and they're serving eggnog, have a glass if it's alcohol-free and pasteurized.
~ Raw fruits and vegetables can be very satisfying.
~ Avoid raw seafood and/or meat and soft cheeses, such as Brie, Camembert and feta. They may contain the bacteria that cause listeriosis.

Adding 300 Calories

Around week 13 or 14 of your pregnancy (the end of the 1st trimester), you'll probably need to start adding an extra 300 calories to your meal plan to meet the needs of your growing fetus and your changing body. Below are some choices of extra food for one day to get those 300 calories.

- Choice #1: 2 thin slices pork, ½ cup cabbage, 1 carrot
- Choice #2: ½ cup cooked brown rice, ¾ cup strawberries, 1 cup orange juice, 1 slice fresh pineapple
- Choice #3: 4-ounce salmon steak, 1 cup asparagus, 2 cups Romaine lettuce
- Choice #4: 1 cup cooked pasta, 1 slice fresh tomato, 1 cup of 1% milk, ½ cup cooked green beans, ¼ cantaloupe

---

My husband and I eat out a lot because we're tired after work. Are there any foods I should avoid at restaurants?

It's OK to eat out at restaurants; just be careful about what you eat. Avoid any raw meats or raw seafood. If some foods don't agree with you at home, avoid them when you eat out. Chicken or fish, clear soups, fresh fruits and vegetables, and salads are usually your best bets. Be careful with calorie-loaded salad dressings, fat-laden sauces, adding butter or piling on sour cream, if excessive weight gain is a concern. Avoid highly spicy foods or foods that contain a lot of sodium, such as some Chinese food.

A Week of Sample Meal Plans for Pregnancy (for Normal-Weight Women)

DAY 1
Breakfast
>   1 cup high-fiber cereal
>   1 cup milk
>   1 medium piece of fruit

Snack
>   1 small muffin

Lunch
>   2 cups dark leafy lettuce
>   ½ cup garbanzo beans
>   1 hard-cooked egg
>   2 T lowfat salad dressing
>   1 slice whole-wheat bread
>   1 cup milk

Snack
>   1 medium piece of fruit
>   1 ounce roasted nuts

Dinner
    4 ounces baked chicken
    1 cup brown rice
    1 cup steamed broccoli
    1 cup tomato juice
Snack
    6 graham cracker pieces (4 pieces make one whole cracker)
    1 cup milk

DAY 2
Breakfast
    1 egg, scrambled
    1 slice toast
    1 T margarine
    1 cup calcium-fortified orange juice
Snack
    1 peach or apple
Lunch
    1 cup soup
    1 ounce hard cheese
    6 crackers
    1 glass water with lemon
    8 ounces yogurt
Snack
    assorted raw veggies
    ¼ cup low-cal dip
Dinner
    4 ounces orange roughy
    1 medium potato
    2 T lowfat or fatfree sour cream
    1 cup veggies

   1 cup milk
Snack
   2 Fig Newtons
   1 cup vegetable or fruit juice

DAY 3
Breakfast
   1 waffle
   1 T syrup
   1 cup decaf coffee
   ½ cup fruit
Snack
   ½ English muffin
   1 T jam
Lunch
   2 slices whole-wheat bread
   1½ ounces cooked chicken
   1 T lowfat mayonnaise
   tomato-and-lettuce salad
   lemon juice for salad
   1 cup milk
Snack
   6 whole-wheat crackers
   2 T humus
Dinner
   4 ounces lean pork, fat removed
   ¾ cup cooked pasta
   1 T margarine for pasta
   sliced tomatoes
   1 small roll
   1 glass water with lemon

Snack
>½ cup pudding
>3 vanilla wafers

DAY 4
Breakfast
>1 medium bagel
>2 T peanut butter
>1 cup chocolate milk
>1 piece of fruit

Snack
>½ cup yogurt
>2 T granola

Lunch
>1 slice pita bread
>2 hard-cooked eggs, mashed
>3 T lowfat mayonnaise to make egg salad
>1 cup salad greens and fixings
>2 T lowfat dressing
>1 cup milk

Snack
>2 celery stalks
>3 T cream cheese

Dinner
>1 medium portion of lasagna
>1 serving antipasto
>1 slice garlic bread
>1 glass water with lemon

Snack
>½ cup lowfat ice cream
>2 macaroons

DAY 5

Breakfast
   1 fruit-and-yogurt smoothie
   1 medium banana-nut muffin
Snack
   ½ cup lowfat cottage cheese
   1 small orange, cut into chunks
Lunch
   1½ cups vegetable soup
   1 whole-wheat roll
   2 ounces lowfat cheese
   1 cup milk
Snack
   ⅓ cup bean dip
   5 whole-wheat crackers
Dinner
   4 ounces beef steak
   1 medium sweet potato
   1 T margarine for potato
   1 cup mixed vegetables
   1 glass water with lemon
Snack
   1 ounce cheddar cheese
   3 crackers

DAY 6

Breakfast
   1 cup oatmeal
   1 T brown sugar for oatmeal
   1 cup orange juice

Snack
>   1 cup fresh vegetables, assorted
>   ¼ cup lowfat spinach dip

Lunch
>   1 cup shredded lowfat cheese
>   1 whole-wheat flour 10-inch tortilla (melt cheese on tortilla, then wrap and eat)
>   1 cup tomato soup
>   1 cup milk

Snack
>   6 whole-wheat crackers
>   2 T guacamole

Dinner
>   4-ounce turkey burger
>   1 whole-wheat bun
>   condiments for burger
>   1 cup baked potato fries
>   1 medium corn on the cob
>   1 T margarine for corn
>   1 glass water with lemon

Snack
>   1 cup gelatin dessert, with 2 T lowfat whipped topping
>   3 chocolate cookies

DAY 7

Breakfast
>   3 small pancakes
>   1½ T syrup
>   1 cup grapefruit juice
>   ½ cup yogurt

Snack
   1 medium blueberry muffin
   1 small tangerine
Lunch
   2 slices whole-wheat bread
   ½ can tuna, packed in water
   2 T lowfat mayonnaise for sandwich
   tomato and lettuce for sandwich
   6 potato chips
   1 cup milk
Snack
   ½ peanut butter sandwich
   2 T raisins
Dinner
   4 ounces chicken
   1 cup pasta salad
   1 cup green beans
   sliced tomatoes
   1 small roll
   1 glass water with lemon
Snack
   ½ bagel
   2 T cream cheese

Eating Wisely at the End of Pregnancy

Toward the end of your pregnancy, you may find you have
a harder time with your food plan than you had earlier in

pregnancy. You may be bored with the foods you've been eating.

End-of-Pregnancy
Foods to Eat, Amounts and Serving Sizes

The list below can help you focus on the amounts of food you need for the last part of your pregnancy.

Breads, cereals, rice, pasta and grains—*at least 6 servings*—1 slice of bread, ½ bun, ½ English muffin or bagel, ½ cup cooked pasta, rice or hot cereal, 4 crackers, ½ cup cooked cereal

Fruit—*2 to 4 servings*—¼ cup dried fruit, ½ cup fresh, canned or cooked fruit, ¾ cup juice

Vegetables—*4 servings*—½ cup cooked vegetables, 1 cup leafy salad vegetables, ¾ cup juice, 1 medium potato

Protein sources—*2 to 4 servings*—2 to 4 ounces of cooked poultry, meat or fish, ½ to 1 cup cooked beans, 1 ounce seeds or nuts, ½ cup tofu, 1 egg

Dairy products—*4 servings*—1 cup milk (any type), 1 cup yogurt, 1 to 1½ ounces cheese, ¾ cup cottage cheese, ½ cup frozen yogurt or ice cream

Fats, oils and sweets—limit intake of these food products and concentrate on nutritious, healthy foods

---

Your baby is getting larger, and you don't seem to have as much room for food now. Heartburn and/or indigestion may also be problems for you. But don't give up on good nutrition!

- It's important to continue to pay attention to what you eat so you can continue to provide your baby the healthful nutrition it needs before its birth.
- Every day, try to eat one serving of a dark leafy vegetable, a serving of food or juice rich in vitamin C and one serving of a food high in vitamin A (many foods that are yellow/orange, such as yams, carrots and cantaloupes, are good sources of vitamin A).
- Remember to keep up your fluid intake.

When Labor Begins

- A woman often gets nauseated when she's in labor, which may cause vomiting.
- For your health and comfort, your doctor wants to avoid this problem, so you will be advised to keep your stomach empty during labor for your own safety.
- You probably won't be interested in eating, but you may be very thirsty. You won't be allowed to drink anything during labor for the same reasons as stated above.
- You may, however, be allowed sips of water or ice chips to suck on. You may even be offered a wet face cloth to suck on to relieve your thirst.

- If your labor is long, your body may be hydrated with fluids through an I.V.
- After your baby's birth, if everything is OK, you will be able to eat and drink.

If You're Planning to Breastfeed Your Baby

After birth, your body continues to need lots of vitamins and minerals for your growing baby—you'll need even more of them if you choose to breastfeed!

- It's important to realize how necessary your continued good nutrition is for you and your baby.
- If you're going to breastfeed baby, you need to begin thinking about nutritional needs for the time you will nurse.
- A breastfeeding mother secretes 425 to 700 calories into her breast milk *every day!*
- You will probably be advised to eat about 500 calories extra each day during this time.
- The extra calories you take in help you maintain your own good health. These calories should also be nutritious and healthy, like the ones you've been eating during pregnancy.

- You may have to avoid some foods because they can pass into breast milk and cause stomach distress in your baby.
- Avoid chocolate, foods that produce gas in you, such as Brussels sprouts and cauliflower, highly spiced foods and any other foods you have problems with.
- Discuss the situation with your doctor and your pediatrician if you have questions.
- In addition to the food you eat, you need to drink lots of fluids.
- You need to drink at least 2 quarts of fluid (that's right—you need to keep on drinking water!) every day to make enough milk for your baby and to stay hydrated. You'll need more in hot weather.
- Avoid caffeine-containing drinks because caffeine can pass to your baby through your breast milk.
- Although caffeine is out of your bloodstream in 3 to 5 hours, it can remain in a baby's bloodstream for up to 96 hours!
- Keep up your calcium intake; it's very important if you breastfeed.
- Ask your doctor about vitamin supplements.
- Some mothers continue taking their prenatal vitamin as long as they breastfeed.

Breastfeeding Needs

This chart shows your daily requirements during breastfeeding.

Vitamins & Minerals	Needs During Breastfeeding
A	1300mcg
B_1 (thiamine)	1.6mg
B_2 (riboflavin)	1.8mg
B_3 (niacin)	20mg
B_6	2.2mg
B_{12}	2.6mcg
C	95mg
Calcium	1200mg
D	10mcg
E	12mg
Folic acid	280mcg
Iron	15mg
Magnesium	355mg
Phosphorus	1200mg
Zinc	19mg

Nutrition after Pregnancy

After birth, you need to add an extra 500 calories to your normal diet if you breastfeed. Below are some tips for getting what you need.

- To save valuable time and effort, buy prepackaged or semiprepared foods, such as cleaned, precut fruits and vegetables.

- Keep eating five or six small meals a day.
- Eat for energy—whole-grain products and protein are good choices. Avoid sugar; it can make you feel tired.
- Now is not the time to diet, but you can choose low-fat foods. Also eat plenty of fruits and vegetables to help fill you up.
- Keep drinking a lot of water, whether you breastfeed or bottlefeed.
- Limit coffee or tea intake to one cup a day if you breastfeed to avoid passing caffeine to baby.
- Some smart snacks that may add some variety to your after-birth nutrition plan include the following:
  - ~ cold gazpacho soup on a hot day
  - ~ half a cantaloupe filled with fresh berries sprinkled with 1 tablespoon of wheat germ and 1 teaspoon of sugar or a packet of Splenda
  - ~ ½ cup prepared humus with fresh veggies or low-salt crackers
  - ~ ½ cup salsa mixed with 2 tablespoons of diced avocado, served with ½ cup baked tortilla chips or low-salt crackers
  - ~ fruit smoothie made with ½ cup plain or flavored lowfat or fatfree yogurt, 6 ounces of calcium-fortified orange juice and half a banana or a handful of berries

A Week of Sample
Meal Plans for Breastfeeding

Nutrition for a nursing mother needs to be high quality, but it should taste good, too! The foods listed below supply you with the nutrition you need to help you make breast milk and to give you energy.

DAY 1
Breakfast
    1 egg, scrambled or poached
    2 slices toast
    1 T margarine
    ½ grapefruit or cantaloupe
    1 cup milk
Midmorning Snack
    1 cup tea
    1 cup grapes
    2 crackers
Lunch
    2 cups salad
    2 T light salad dressing
    2 slices bread
    1 slice lowfat American or Swiss cheese
    1 piece of fruit, such as an apple or a pear
    1 cup water
Midafternoon Snack
    1 slice of raisin toast
    1 T margarine
    1 ounce hard cheese
    ½ cup fruit

Dinner
   1 small chicken breast
   1½ cups sautéed fresh vegetables
   ²/₃ cup brown rice
   sliced tomatoes
   1 cup water
Snack
   4 ounces yogurt
   4 small crackers

DAY 2
Breakfast
   ½ to 1 cup cereal
   ½ cup milk for cereal
   1 slice toast
   1 T jam or jelly
   ¾ cup calcium-fortified orange juice
Midmorning Snack
   1 medium orange
   ½ ounce of nuts
Lunch
   1 slice meat-and-cheese pizza
   ¾ cup fruit salad
   1 cup milk
Midafternoon Snack
   ½ cup cottage cheese
   1 medium apple, cut into small chunks
   1 t cinnamon
   sugar or Splenda to taste
Dinner
   4 ounces pork, fat removed

¾ cup cooked vegetables, such as corn or peas
1 medium baked potato
1 T margarine or 2 T fatfree sour cream for potato
1 slice whole-wheat bread
1 cup water
Snack
½ cup pudding
2 small cookies

DAY 3
Breakfast
3 medium pancakes
2 T syrup
orange slices
1 cup decaf coffee
Midmorning Snack
½ cup cottage cheese
2 fresh pineapple rings
Lunch
2 slices whole-wheat toast
1½ ounces deli meat
1 T mayonnaise
lettuce and tomato
1 cup milk
Midafternoon Snack
¾ cup pudding
¼ cup nonfat or lowfat whipped topping
Dinner
4 ounces red snapper
2 cups lettuce
tomato wedges

2 T lowfat dressing
⅓ cup risotto
1 small roll
1 cup water
Snack
4 vanilla wafers
1 cup lowfat cocoa

DAY 4
Breakfast
1-egg omelet
2 ounces shredded cheese
1 slice toast
1 T margarine
1 cup grapefruit juice
Midmorning Snack
1 cup herbal tea
1 cup strawberries
2 small cookies
Lunch
1 cup shredded cheese
2 small flour tortillas (melt ½ cheese on each tortilla, wrap and eat)
1 cup salad
2 T salad dressing
1 cup water
Midafternoon Snack
1 slice of whole-wheat toast
1 T margarine
¼ cup cottage cheese
½ cup fruit

Dinner
> 1 serving of spaghetti and meatballs
> 1 cup minestrone soup
> 1 slice sourdough bread
> 1 T margarine
> 1 cup milk

Snack
> 1 frozen fruit bar

DAY 5

Breakfast
> 1 large waffle
> 2 T syrup for waffle
> ¾ cup calcium-fortified orange juice

Midmorning Snack
> 1 pomegranate
> 4 vegetable crackers

Lunch
> 1½ cups chicken-with-rice soup
> 6 whole-wheat crackers
> 1 ounce hard cheese
> 1 cup lemonade

Midafternoon Snack
> 1 cup gelatin dessert
> 1 medium pear

Dinner
> 2 medium tacos
> 1 cup Spanish rice
> ⅓ cup guacamole
> ½ cup mild salsa

    1 medium salad
    1 cup milk
Snack
    ½ cup frozen yogurt
    2 T lowfat whipped topping

DAY 6
Breakfast
    1 cup oatmeal
    2 T brown sugar for oatmeal
    ½ cup milk
    1 medium apple
    1 cup decaf coffee
Midmorning Snack
    ½ cup tapioca pudding
    2 small macaroons
Lunch
    2 slices whole-wheat toast
    ½ can water-packed tuna
    2 T mayonnaise
    lettuce and tomato
    6 potato chips
    1 cup milk
Midafternoon Snack
    ¾ cup yogurt
    ¼ cup granola
Dinner
    4 ounces lamb
    1 cup pasta
    2 T margarine for pasta

1 cup mixed vegetables
1 small roll
1 cup milk
Snack
½ cup trail mix
1 cup orange juice

DAY 7
Breakfast
1 medium bagel
2 T cream cheese
2 slices bacon
1 cup apple juice
Midmorning Snack
½ cup lowfat ice cream
¼ cup berries
Lunch
2 slices cheese pizza
lettuce and tomato salad
1 cup milk
Midafternoon Snack
1½ ounces cheddar cheese
4 whole-wheat crackers
Dinner
4 ounces beef steak
1 cup oven-baked ranch fries
1 medium corn on the cob
1 small roll
1 cup milk
Snack
½ peanut butter sandwich
1 cup cranberry juice

A Week of Sample
Meal Plans for Bottlefeeding

A day's nutrition for a bottlefeeding mother is different from that of a woman who breastfeeds. You don't need to consume as many calories, and your fluid intake doesn't need to be as high.

DAY 1

Breakfast
    1 cup cereal
    1 T sugar or Splenda
    1 cup milk
Midmorning Snack
    ½ cup peaches
    ½ cup milk
    1 cereal bar
Lunch
    2 cups salad
    2 T light salad dressing
    2 slices bread
    1 slice lowfat cheese
    1 piece of fruit, such as an apple or pear
Midafternoon Snack
    1 slice of toast
    4 ounces skim milk
    1 small piece of fruit
Dinner
    4 ounces salmon
    ¾ cup rice
    1 cup salad
    1 T salad dressing

sliced veggie assortment

1 cup water

Snack

1 whole graham cracker (4 squares in one cracker)

¾ cup orange juice

DAY 2

Breakfast

½ toasted English muffin

1 T peanut butter

4 ounces cottage cheese

Midmorning Snack

8 ounces yogurt

2 fatfree cookies

Lunch

grilled cheese sandwich (2 slices whole-wheat toast and
2 slices fatfree or lowfat cheese)

sliced tomatoes

1 pickle

1 cup coffee

Midafternoon Snack

½ cup tapioca

2 small cookies

Dinner

4 ounces chicken breast

½ cup vegetables

1 slice whole-wheat bread

sliced tomatoes

8 ounces water

Snack

1 cup instant fatfree cocoa

1 small cookie

DAY 3
Breakfast
    1 serving of oatmeal
    1 T brown sugar
    1 cup milk
    ½ cup cranberry juice
Midmorning Snack
    1 English muffin
    2 T sugarfree jam or jelly
Lunch
    2 small fatfree flour tortillas
    1 cup fatfree refried beans
    ⅓ cup salsa
    ⅓ cup fatfree cheddar cheese
    1 plum or peach
Midafternoon Snack
    1 cup tomato juice
    4 whole-wheat crackers
Dinner
    4 ounces roast beef
    1 medium potato
    ¼ cup fatfree sour cream
    1 cup mixed vegetables
    1 small roll
    1 cup water with lemon
Snack
    8 ounces yogurt
    handful of grapes

DAY 4

Breakfast
1 cup grits or farina
1 T margarine
1 cup milk

Midmorning Snack
1 small apple
½ cup chocolate milk

Lunch
1 beef taco
⅓ cup fatfree refried beans
1 piece of watermelon

Midafternoon Snack
1 cup vegetable juice
3 rye crackers

Dinner
1 serving chili
½ cup rice
1 cup green peas
1 slice garlic bread
1 cup water with lemon

Snack
½ cup fatfree frozen yogurt
2 T chocolate syrup

DAY 5

Breakfast
1 small bagel
2 T lowfat flavored cream cheese
1 cup grapefruit juice

Midmorning Snack
> ½ cup tapioca pudding
> 2 macaroons

Lunch
> 1 cup brown rice
> 2 ounces cooked chicken
> 1 T soy sauce
> 1 cup cooked vegetables
> 1 cup coffee

Midafternoon Snack
> 1 cup fatfree gelatin
> ½ cup grapes

Dinner
> 4 ounces oven-fried chicken
> 1 medium baked potato
> 2 T fatfree sour cream
> 1 cup steamed broccoli
> 1 small roll
> 8 ounces water

Snack
> 1 cup hot apple cider
> 2 graham crackers

DAY 6

Breakfast
> 1 egg, scrambled or fried
> 1 piece whole-wheat toast
> 1 T jam or jelly
> 1 cup milk
> ½ cup cranberry/apple juice

Midmorning Snack
   2 minibagels
   1 T peanut butter
Lunch
   1 veggie patty
   1 whole-wheat bun
   condiments for the burger
   5 baked potato chips
   1 cup skim milk
   1 nectarine
Midafternoon Snack
   1 slice of cinnamon toast
   4 ounces skim milk
   ½ cup cantaloupe chunks
Dinner
   1 serving enchilada casserole
   1 cup corn
   1 cup Spanish rice
   ¼ cup fatfree sour cream
   1 cup water with lemon
Snack
   ⅔ cup fatfree ice cream
   handful of fresh berries

DAY 7
Breakfast
   2 medium pancakes
   2 T light syrup
   1 cup skim milk
   ½ cup prune juice

Midmorning Snack
> ⅓ cup trail mix
> 1 cup fatfree hot cocoa

Lunch
> 1½ cups tomato bisque soup
> 5 whole-wheat crackers
> 1 ounce cheddar cheese
> 1 cup mixed berries

Midafternoon Snack
> 1 cup pineapple juice
> 4 whole-wheat crackers

Dinner
> 4 ounces lean pork, fat removed
> ⅔ cup sweet-potato casserole
> 1 T margarine
> 1 cup green beans
> 1 small roll
> 1 cup skim milk

Snack
> 8 ounces yogurt
> 2 small ginger snap cookies

Part III: Weight Management

How Much Weight Should I Gain?

Every woman needs to gain a certain amount of weight during pregnancy. Proper weight gain helps ensure you and your baby are healthy at the time of delivery.

Today, recommendations for weight gain during pregnancy are higher than they were in the past; normal weight gain is 25 to 35 pounds. If you are underweight at the start of your pregnancy, expect to gain between 28 and 40 pounds. If you're overweight before pregnancy, you probably should not gain as much weight. Acceptable weight gain is between 15 and 25 pounds. Recommendations vary, so discuss the matter with your doctor. Eat nutritious, well-balanced meals during your pregnancy. Do *not* diet now!

Many years ago, women were not allowed to gain much weight—sometimes only 12 to 15 pounds for an entire pregnancy! Today, we know that restricting weight gain to this extent is not healthy for the baby or the mother-to-be. But don't go overboard, either, just because you're pregnant.

You may be eating for two, but you don't have to eat twice as much!

- As an average for a normal-weight woman, many doctors suggest a weight gain of $2/3$ of a pound (10 ounces) a week until 20 weeks, then 1 pound a week through the 40th week. This recommendation is *only* an average; actual suggestions vary according to your needs.
- It isn't unusual not to gain weight or even to lose a little weight early in pregnancy.
- Your doctor will keep careful track of changes in your weight. You should watch your weight, but don't be obsessive about it.
- Gain weight slowly.
- If you're in good shape when you get pregnant, with an appropriate amount of body fat, and if you exercise regularly and eat healthfully, you should not have a problem with excessive weight gain.
- Getting on the scale and seeing your weight rise may be very hard for you. Tell yourself it's OK to gain weight.
- You don't have to let yourself go—you can control your weight by eating nutritiously. But you need to gain enough weight to meet the needs of your pregnancy.

I have such a fear of getting fat during pregnancy, I know it's going to cause me a lot of problems. What can I do about it?

You must be prepared to gain weight while you're pregnant. It's a normal part of pregnancy and necessary for your baby's health! Getting on the scale and seeing your weight increase can be hard, especially if you've had to watch your weight closely. You must decide at the beginning of your pregnancy that it's OK to gain weight—it's for the good health of your baby. You can control your weight gain by eating carefully and nutritiously; you don't have to gain an extra 50 pounds. But you must gain enough weight to meet the needs of your pregnancy.

Increasing Your Caloric Intake

- During the 1st trimester (first 13 weeks), you should eat a total of about 2200 calories a day.
- During the 2nd and 3rd trimesters, you probably need an additional 300 calories each day.
- These extra calories provide the energy your body needs for you and your growing baby.

- Be cautious about adding the extra 300 calories to your nutrition plan—it doesn't mean doubling your portions.
- A medium apple and a cup of lowfat yogurt add up to 300 calories!
- Some women need more calories; some women need fewer. If you are underweight when you begin pregnancy, you will probably have to eat more than 300 extra calories each day. If you're overweight, you may have less need for extra calories.
- It can be unhealthy for you and your baby if you gain too much weight during pregnancy.
- The key to good nutrition and weight management is to eat a balanced diet throughout your pregnancy.
- Eat the foods you need to help your baby grow and develop.
- Your baby uses the nutrients it receives to create and to store protein, fat and carbohydrates. It also needs energy for fetal body processes to function.
- Extra calories support the changes your body is going through. For example, your uterus increases in size and your blood volume increases by about 50%.
- Calories aren't interchangeable. You can't eat whatever you want and expect to get the best nutrition

for your baby and you; eating right takes care and attention.

- You need to eat foods high in vitamins and minerals, especially iron, calcium, magnesium, folic acid and zinc.
- Eating a wide variety of foods each day can supply you with the nutrients you need. Choose from dairy products, protein foods, fruits and vegetables, and breads and cereals.
- Avoid junk food and foods loaded with empty calories.
- Choose your foods wisely.
- For example, if you're overweight, avoid high-calorie peanut butter and other nuts as a protein source; instead choose lowfat cheese, fatfree yogurt and other lowfat products.
- If you're underweight, high-calorie ice cream and milkshakes are acceptable dairy sources.

Do I really need to increase the number of calories I eat, now that I'm pregnant?

Yes. Most experts agree a normal-weight pregnant woman needs to increase her caloric intake by at least 300 calories a day during the 2nd and 3rd trimesters. These extra calories are important for tissue growth in you and your baby. Your baby is using the energy from your calories to create and to store protein, fat and carbohydrates, and to provide energy for its own body processes.

When You're Overweight

If you are overweight when you get pregnant, you're not alone. Statistics show that up to 38% of all pregnant

---

Where Does the Weight Go?

A weight gain of 25 to 35 pounds may sound like a lot when the baby only weighs about 7 pounds; however, weight is distributed between you and your baby. Weight gained during pregnancy is normally distributed as shown in the chart below.

Distribution of Weight Gained during Pregnancy

Weight	Location
7½ pounds	Baby
14 pounds	Maternal stores (fat, protein and other nutrients)
4 pounds	Increased fluid volume
2 pounds	Uterus
2 pounds	Amniotic fluid
2 pounds	Breast enlargement
1½ pounds	Placenta

women fall into this category. You are considered over-weight if your body mass index (BMI) is between 25 and 30; over 30, you are considered obese. Ask your doctor to help you figure out your BMI at a prenatal appointment. Or do it yourself using the formula in the box on page 131.

- Being overweight brings special challenges. When you're overweight, pregnancy and delivery can be harder on you.
- Try to gain your 15 to 25 pounds of total-pregnancy weight *slowly*.
- Aim for a weight gain of 2 to 4 pounds the 1st trimester, 5 to 7 pounds the 2nd trimester and 8 to 14 pounds the 3rd trimester.
- Weigh yourself weekly, and watch your food intake.
- Eat nutritious, healthful foods, and eliminate those with empty calories. The quality of the food you eat is more important than ever when you are pregnant.
- Talk to your doctor about making exercise part of your daily routine. Discuss swimming and walking, which are good exercises for *any* pregnant woman.
- A visit with a nutritionist may be necessary to help you develop a healthful food plan.
- To get your 1200mg of calcium each day, choose nonfat, lowfat and skim dairy products.

- To get the other nutrients you need, choose nonfat or lowfat products, meats, grain products, fruits and vegetables. Many supply a variety of nutrients.
- Take your prenatal vitamin every day throughout your entire pregnancy.
- To get enough fiber, choose whole-wheat carbohydrate sources, and eat lots of fruits and vegetables, without adding sugar to fruits or butter to veggies.
- Eat regular meals—5 to 6 *small* meals a day is a good goal. This helps maintain blood sugar levels and helps with nutrient absorption.
- Your total calorie intake should be between 1800 and 2400 calories a day.
- Keeping a daily food diary helps you keep track of how much you're eating and when you're eating. It can help you identify where to make changes, if they are necessary.
- Give up drinking soda, juices and sweet beverages. Water is best; skim milk and other unsweetened beverages are also good choices.
- You may use Splenda as a sweetener in beverages and with foods.
- Avoid simple sugars, like cake, candy, pie and cookies. Choose complex carbohydrates instead, including fruits, vegetables and whole-grain breads and cereals.

- Learn to make substitutions so you can still enjoy flavorful foods but save on calories. Some choices include those below.
  - ~ Instead of a tuna-salad sandwich with mayonnaise, eat a turkey sandwich with mustard. You'll save 350 calories and 37 grams of fat.
  - ~ Instead of a chef's salad with thousand island dressing, choose a chicken Caesar salad, and leave off the dressing. You'll save 570 calories and 60 grams of fat.
  - ~ Instead of a bagel with cream cheese, opt for an English muffin with lowfat margarine. You'll save 350 calories and 16 grams of fat.

Figuring Your Body Mass Index (BMI)

BMI is determined from the measurement of height and weight. It is calculated using the following formula:

$$BMI = \frac{weight\ (kg)}{height\ squared\ (meters)}$$

If pounds and inches are used:

$$BMI = \frac{weight\ (pounds) \times 703}{height\ squared\ (inches)}$$

I'm overweight, and I just found out I'm pregnant. How much weight should I gain?

If you're overweight before pregnancy, you probably should not gain as much as other women during pregnancy. Acceptable weight gain is 15 to 25 pounds. This is an individual situation that you should discuss with your doctor. It is important for you to eat nutritious, well-balanced meals during your pregnancy. Do *not* diet! If you're overweight when you begin pregnancy, try to gain your total-pregnancy weight *slowly*.

When You're Underweight

If you are underweight when you begin pregnancy, you also face special challenges. In general, you should expect to gain between 28 and 40 pounds. You may find that if you are underweight you need to gain extra weight during pregnancy. Below are some tips for you to help you reach that goal.

- Don't drink diet sodas or eat low-calorie foods.
- Choose nutritious foods that will help you gain weight, such as cheeses, dried fruits, nuts, avocados, whole milk and ice cream.
- Eat foods with a higher calorie content.

- Try to add nutritious, calorie-rich snacks to your daily menu.
- Avoid junk food with lots of empty calories.
- You may need to do *less* exercise, if you burn too many calories in these activities.
- Eating small, frequent meals may help improve digestion and absorption of nutrients.

I'm pregnant and know I'm underweight. How much should I gain during my pregnancy?

If you start your pregnancy underweight, the normal weight gain is 28 to 40 pounds. It's important for you to eat regularly and to eat nutritiously, even if you are not used to doing this.

Target Weight Gain with Multiples

The target weight gain for women carrying more than one baby is quite a bit higher than that for women carrying one baby.

- The desirable weight gain for women expecting twins is about 45 pounds.
- If you are carrying triplets or more, your doctor will advise you how much weight you should gain during your pregnancy.

- Studies show that if a woman gains the targeted amount of weight with a multiple pregnancy, her babies are often healthier.
- Usually women who gain the targeted amount of weight during pregnancy lose it after delivery.
- One study showed that women who gained the suggested amount of weight during a twin pregnancy were close to their prepregnant weight 2 years after delivery.
- When you consider the average size of the babies (about 5 to 6 pounds each) and the weight of the placenta(s) (1½ pounds for each), plus the weight of the additional amniotic fluid, you can see where the extra weight goes.

How am I supposed to watch my weight gain and still eat more calories every day?

Not every woman needs to increase her food intake by 300 calories; that's just a general guideline. You must look at your individual case. If you're underweight when you begin pregnancy, you may have to eat more than 300 extra calories each day. If you're overweight when you get pregnant, you may have less need for those extra calories. The key to good nutrition and weight management is to eat a balanced diet throughout your entire pregnancy. Eat the foods you need to help your baby grow and develop, but choose wisely.

Super Hawaiian Smoothie

1 8-ounce can chunk pineapple, packed in its own juice
1 cup calcium-fortified citrus juice
1 cup fatfree or lowfat flavored yogurt
Freeze pineapple in the can until frozen. Run warm water over can for a few minutes before opening. In a blender, place juice and yogurt, then add pineapple. Scoop out pineapple with an ice-cream scoop. Blend all ingredients on high until smooth.

Eating Disorders— Can They Affect Pregnancy?

If you believe you have an eating disorder, try to deal with it *before* you get pregnant! Problems associated with an eating disorder during pregnancy include the following:

- a low-birthweight baby
- a weight gain during pregnancy that is *too low*
- increased chance of fetal death
- low 5-minute Apgar scores
- intrauterine-growth restriction
- baby in a breech presentation (because it may be born too early)

- high blood pressure in the mother-to-be
- miscarriage
- birth defects
- electrolyte problems in the mother-to-be
- decreased plasma volume

If you have an eating disorder, talk to your doctor about the problem as soon as possible. It is serious and can affect both you and your baby.

Helpful Hints for
Watching Your Calories

- If you're watching your calorie intake, you might choose lowfat or fatfree foods to help you cut back on calories.
- They can be a good choice, but they won't help you if you eat too much of them because they still contain calories—sometimes lots of them!
- Many pregnant women believe the kind of food they eat matters more than the amount they eat, so they eat more.
- In many cases, a pregnant woman eats more calories than she normally would! Don't make this mistake.

My doctor said I must get weighed each time I come in. Can't I just weigh myself at home before I come in and tell the doctor or nurse my weight?

It's best to be weighed at the office. Your doctor needs to know how your weight is changing, and getting weighed on the same scale (at the office) is the best way to do that. Your weight change is one way your doctor can tell that everything is progressing normally with your pregnancy. Although you may be shy about being weighed, it's an important part of your visit to the doctor. Your healthcare team is doing it to make sure everything is OK with your pregnancy.

Weight Changes after Baby's Birth

Don't get anxious about losing pregnancy weight after your baby's birth. Regaining your prepregnancy figure may take longer than you hope it will.

- It's normal to lose 10 to 15 pounds immediately after your baby is born.
- You may retain 5 pounds of fluid, but it washes out of your system within a few days.

- Extra weight may be harder to lose.
- Your body stores about 7 to 10 pounds of fat as energy for the first few months after birth. If you eat properly and get enough exercise, these pounds will slowly come off.
- If you breastfeed, all the nutrients your baby receives depend on the quality of the food you eat.
- Breastfeeding places more demands on your body than pregnancy. Your body burns up to 700 calories a day just to produce milk.
- When breastfeeding, you need to eat an extra 500 calories a day. Be sure they're nutritious calories (eat fruits, vegetables and breads—stay away from junk food).
- Keep up fluid levels, too, when you breastfeed.
- See the week of sample meal plans for breastfeeding moms that begins on page 108.

Also by Glade B. Curtis, M.D., M.P.H., OB/GYN and Judith Schuler, M.S.

Your Pregnancy
Week by Week, 5th Edition
ISBN: 1-55561-346-2 (paper)
1-55561-347-0 (cloth)

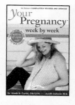

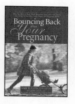

Bouncing Back
After Your Pregnancy
ISBN: 0-7382-0606-7

Your Baby's First Year,
Week by Week
ISBN: 1-55561-232-6 (paper)
1-55561-257-1 (cloth)

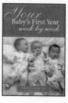

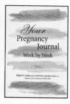

Your Pregnancy Journal
Week by Week
ISBN: 1-55561-343-8

Your Pregnancy
for the Father to Be
ISBN: 1-55561-345-4

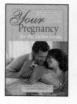

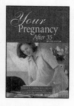

Your Pregnancy After 35
ISBN: 1-55561-319-5

Your Pregnancy
Questions and Answers
ISBN: 0-7382-1003-X

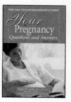

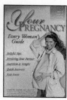

Your Pregnancy:
Every Woman's Guide
ISBN: 0-7382-1001-3

Da Capo Lifelong Books are available wherever books are sold and at special discounts for bulk purchases in the U.S. by corporations, institutions, and other organizations. For more information, please contact the Special Markets Department at the Perseus Books Group, 11 Cambridge Center, Cambridge, MA 02142, or call (800) 255-1514, or e-mail special.markets@perseusbooks.com.